Group B Strep Explained

Dr Sara Wickham

Group B Strep Explained
Second edition published 2019 by Birthmoon Creations
Avebury, Wiltshire
© 2019 Sara Wickham
www.sarawickham.com

Sara Wickham has asserted her moral right to be named as the author of this work in accordance with the Copyright, Designs and Patents Act of 1988.

ISBN-10: 1999806425
ISBN-13: 978-1999806422
Also available as an e-book

Cover design by Chris Hackforth

This book offers general information for interest only and does not constitute or replace individualised professional midwifery or medical care and advice. Whilst every effort has been made to ensure the accuracy and currency of the information herein, the author accepts no liability or responsibility for any loss or damage caused, or thought to be caused, by making decisions based upon the information in this book and recommends that you use it in conjunction with other trusted sources of information.

About the Author

Dr Sara Wickham PhD, RM, MA, PGCert, BA(Hons) is a midwife, educator, writer and researcher who works independently, dividing her working time between speaking, writing, teaching online courses and live workshops, consulting and creating resources for midwives and birth workers.

Sara's career has been varied; she has lived and worked in the UK, the USA and New Zealand, edited three professional journals and lectured in more than twenty-five countries.

You can find Sara online at www.sarawickham.com, where she writes a twice weekly blog and a free monthly newsletter. Some of her work is also shared at www.facebook.com/saramidwife and @DrSaraWickham

Also by Sara Wickham

Anti-D in Midwifery: panacea or paradox?
Appraising Research into Childbirth
Birthing Your Placenta (with Nadine Edwards)
Inducing Labour: making informed decisions
Midwifery Best Practice (volumes 1-5)
Sacred Cycles: the spiral of women's wellbeing
Vitamin K and the Newborn
What's Right for Me? Making decisions in pregnancy and childbirth
101 Tips for planning, writing and surviving your dissertation

Acknowledgements

To the women and families whose questions and desire for respectful, woman-centred maternity care has always fuelled my practice, research, teaching and writing, thank you. Although this book features the words of just a few (with permission, of course), I am grateful to all of those who question and seek out the best for themselves and their family. This book also contains the words of midwives and obstetricians who shared their experiences, stories and viewpoints in order to broaden the perspectives that this book offers, and I am hugely grateful to each of them for their input.

As ever, the birth of this book has been facilitated by an amazing team of midwives, birth activists, childbirth educators, doctors and friends. Special thanks for help with this edition go to Beverley Beech, Gill Boden, Nadine Edwards, Julie Frohlich, Chris Hackforth, Rachel Reed and Kirsten Small, who all helped it become better through their reading, editing, comments, suggestions and reference wizardry. Thanks also to the rest of my colleagues in the Birth Practice and Politics Forum who have supported me through the publication of many of my books: Sarah Davies, Mavis Kirkham, Jo Murphy-Lawless, Jean Robinson, Helen Shallow and Vicki Williams.

And thank you also to those of you who will buy this book (sometimes repeatedly, I know, because some people will enter a postnatal haze and forget to return it) in order to enable more women and families to think about these important issues. I'm always delighted when my work can help you in yours, and I so appreciate your support, questions and thoughts which help me to write books that will be useful.

Contents

Introduction

As I write the second edition of this book, I remain aware that this is an incredibly emotive area for some people. Issues relating to Group B strep (GBS) bacteria and early onset group B strep (EOGBS) disease affect only a tiny number of babies, but EOGBS disease can sometimes be fatal for those babies and devastating to their families. Our knowledge about whether and how we might be able to predict and prevent EOGBS disease is only partial, and women and families have to decide between a number of options, none of which are ideal. The best that we can do in the current climate is to offer intravenous antibiotics to tens of thousands of women when they are in labour, but we don't have good evidence that these are effective. We do know that antibiotics have unwanted consequences, both for those women and babies who are exposed to them and for future generations who will suffer if bacteria become resistant to them. For all of these reasons and more, the decisions that women and families need to make in this area are not always easy, and this book is designed to help explain the problem, the issues and the evidence.

In the weeks before I began to write both this book and the previous edition, I invited friends, students, online course participants and colleagues to send me their thoughts and comments on what they would like to see included. I have tried to make sure that I have addressed as many of the questions that I received as possible, even if sometimes the best I can do is to acknowledge the importance of the question and say that we do not know the answer.

The diversity of opinions reflected in the responses that I received did not really surprise me, for I have given many talks on this topic over the past few years and am used to hearing a range of views. But I still want to say a little bit about this before we begin the book proper because, if you are new to this area, I think it may be valuable for you to know that there are some very distinctive and different perspectives on the subject of EOGBS disease and the decisions that people make in relation to it. Also, because I think it is vital for people to understand how information from different sources will be influenced by the experiences, beliefs and opinions of the people offering it, I would like to be very open and honest about how I have approached this book so that you can make your own judgment about the value of this (and hopefully all other) information to you.

Quite a lot of the information that is available online and from group B strep-related organisations is written by people who have either lost babies themselves because of EOGBS disease, or who spend time supporting families who have gone through this. In fact, the authors of one of the most significant medical reviews of this area noted that pressure from parents and the media was a factor in the introduction of guidelines for EOGBS disease prevention (Ohlsson & Shah 2014). It is completely understandable that people who have had tragic experiences want to prevent others from experiencing similar things, and we see this in a number of different areas of maternity care these days but decisions relating to this area are not cut-and-dried. There are multiple dimensions to consider.

When I was writing the first edition of this book, I received a couple of emails from women who had lost babies to EOGBS disease asking if I would tell their stories in full, because they felt that these stories would be more likely to make other women accept (or even demand) the tests and antibiotics that I discuss herein. But I received more than ten times as many requests from women specifically asking me **not** to share such stories because they felt it was unfair to (in their words) *'play the dead baby card'* in order to try to persuade people to accept intervention in a situation where the issues are more complex and less clear than is sometimes portrayed. These women explained that they had felt bullied by other parents, professionals or organisations who were seeking to use emotion to persuade them to take a particular course of action. I have since been thanked by many people for taking this stance, especially since the publication of some rather emotive stories of rare events in some of the literature now recommended to women in the UK.

You still won't find these stories in this book. I have included women's words here and there to illustrate points, but overall I have tried to stick to a fair and reasoned discussion of the issues. That's because I don't think it's appropriate that I or anyone should try and persuade you to take a particular course of action. I cannot possibly know what it is to walk in your shoes, live in your body or grow your baby; we all have to make decisions based on our beliefs, experiences, faith, personal circumstances and/or family situation. Now that you know such stories exist, you can, should you want to, go and look for them – they are not difficult to find and I have signposted a few in the section on women's experiences.

In our culture, you will encounter claims that childbirth is risky and arguments that medical intervention is essential far more often than you will hear the other side of the story. The gist of the other side of this story begins with the assertion that birth is generally a very safe, normal journey but that, no matter what we do, women and babies will occasionally encounter problems such as EOGBS disease. It is policymakers who decide whether to offer screening to try to identify those at higher risk and preventative measures to tens of thousands of women to try to reduce the number of babies who get EOGBS disease. But it is up to each woman to decide whether to accept or decline such measures.

I don't want to only give you one side of the story. I want to try and be as balanced as I can, and give you information from a number of different perspectives so that you can make the decision that is right for you. But in order to do that, I felt I needed to begin by telling you that these different perspectives do exist, and that this book is not just about sharing 'facts' (oh, if only such things existed!) but about unpacking the different perspectives a bit so that you can work out what you think and feel and figure out what that right decision for you, your baby and your family is.

These perspectives go all the way back to the way we think and talk about bacteria, so that's where I am going to begin. Chapter one of this book gives some background and context. I begin with a brief overview of the relationships that we humans have with bacteria and the language that is used to talk about these tiny organisms and the way they affect our bodies and babies. Chapters two and three look at screening and prophylaxis (or preventative measures) for EOGBS disease. Chapter four looks at some of the wider issues, including what happens after a baby is born and chapter five provides easy-to-find answers to questions that women have particularly asked me to address in the book.

I am aware that this book contains some repetition. This is because the issues are complex, and repeating some of the key information can help people make sense of them. Also, not all readers will read this book from cover to cover like a novel; some will need to access information on one element of this issue quickly, or will only be interested in one area or question, yet they still need background information. So please forgive me for wanting to make it easy for those who are more pressed for time.

You will find all the references and details of how you can access further resources at the back of the book. I often write about recent research on this topic, so you might like to visit my website (www.sarawickham.com) and put GBS into the search box and see if there is anything else of interest to you there. If you are a birth professional, I have a free monthly newsletter which you can sign up to in which I update people about new research and thinking and I run online courses on this and related topics which will help you better understand the evidence and communicate it to women and their families.

I hope this book serves you and your family well.

Sara Wickham. Wiltshire, England. Spring 2019.

1. Introducing the issues

Because the issues surrounding GBS bacteria and EOGBS disease are complex, there are some basic terms and concepts that need to be explained before we can really get into discussing the current situation and the research evidence. This chapter introduces some of those key issues and concepts so we can draw upon them in later sections.

A brief introduction to human-bacteria relationships

Bacteria are essential to the continuation of human life. These tiny organisms play a critical role in decomposition, in the making of cheese, yogurt and other fermented dairy products and in all manner of modern technological and industrial processes from the manufacture of drugs to the cleaning up of oil spills.

Human beings also have many bacteria living on and within our bodies. As far as the human body is concerned, individual types of bacteria may be helpful, harmful or benign. In some cases, the nature of a particular kind of bacteria (that is, whether it is helpful, harmful or benign) can change according to circumstances. We actually know very little about this area, although our knowledge is growing quickly. What we do currently know is fascinating, and we are now realising that bacteria are far more important to us and to our survival than we have previously imagined.

For instance, we have within our bodies many helpful bacteria such as the well-known *Lactobacillus acidophilus* which is one of a number of bacteria that help us to digest food. *Lactobacillus acidophilus* can also be used to make yogurt which can be used to treat vaginal infections as well as eaten for nourishment. Because both the bacteria and the human host benefit, the relationship between human beings and *Lactobacillus acidophilus* is described as mutualistic. Indeed, many people are aware that fungal infections such as thrush can become a problem when the bacteria that keep them in check are removed, for instance after someone takes antibiotics.

But not all bacteria are 'friendly'. Well-known examples of bacteria that are usually harmful to the human body include *Salmonella enterica*, *Clostridium tetani*, which causes tetanus, and *Mycobacterium tuberculosis*. The relationship between human and bacteria in these examples is described as parasitic, because the bacteria gain at the expense of their human host. These bacteria may also be described as pathogenic, and the simple definition of a pathogen is something that causes disease.

But sometimes, bacteria appear to live in or on (and thus benefit from) their human host without seeming to be doing anything particularly helpful or harmful. Where this occurs, the relationship between them is described as commensal. In fact, most of the bacteria that live within our bodies are thought to be commensalistic, although it is possible that our assessment of this might change over time as we discover more about some of the bacteria with which we co-exist.

Streptococcus agalactiae, otherwise known as group B streptococcus or GBS, and occasionally referred to as beta strep or haemolytic strep, is considered to be a commensal bacterium. It lives in the gut and/or vagina of around a fifth to a quarter of people in the UK (although, as I will explain below, this figure varies between different geographical areas) and, for most of the time, it minds its own business and neither helps nor harms its host. GBS bacteria can occasionally cause a urine, uterine (womb) or other infection in women, but serious GBS disease in pregnant women is rare. A UK study found that serious GBS disease affected only 1 in about 27,000 women and that 79% of babies born to women who experienced severe sepsis, a life-threatening consequence of infection, did not themselves develop sepsis (Kalin *et al* 2015).

Because they can live in the vagina and the rectum (which is considered an important area of the body when it comes to GBS because it is very close to the vagina), GBS bacteria can be passed to a baby during birth. It is normal and healthy for a baby to pick up its mother's bacteria during birth, and usually this does not cause a problem. Indeed, an increasing amount of scientific evidence shows that this is both necessary and beneficial. We now know that there are significant advantages for a baby to be born vaginally and then breastfed, because both of these things help transmit good bacteria to a baby (Neu & Rushing 2011, Cabrera-Rubio *et al* 2012, Mueller *et al* 2014b, 2015, Stewart *et al* 2018, Zhong *et al* 2019). But occasionally a baby will become sick as a result of picking up GBS bacteria during birth, and, in rare situations, a fatal illness can develop.

Much of the information in this book is about the screening tests and interventions which are offered to pregnant women and women in labour in an attempt to prevent EOGBS disease in babies. Screening tests are used in the hope of determining which babies might be at greater risk of EOGBS disease and prophylactic antibiotics may be offered in an attempt to destroy the bacteria which might cause these babies a problem.

A few notes about language and terminology

One of the things that always comes through loud and clear when I talk to women and their families about the topic of GBS is that some people are upset by the language and terminology used by some professionals and those who lobby for increased GBS screening and prophylaxis.

There are two main problems. Firstly, some people have a tendency to use jargon, often unnecessarily, and this can confuse and complicate decisions. So I am going to try to define and explain every scientific or medical term when it is first used in this book and not to over-use them where a non-scientific term can be used instead.

Let me start as I mean to go on by saying a bit more about some of the terms that I will use often in the book. I mentioned the abbreviations GBS and EOGBS in the introduction. GBS stands for *group B streptococcus* and EOGBS stands for *early-onset group B streptococcus* and that abbreviation is often followed by the word *disease* or occasionally *infection*. I will describe that in more detail below but the key thing to note is that GBS refers to the bacteria and EOGBS disease is the term used to describe the serious infection that occasionally develops in newborn babies who have encountered the GBS bacteria.

Another important word which I will use a lot is *prophylaxis*, which I have already mentioned a few times. The word *prophylaxis* refers to a treatment that is given or an action that is taken in order to prevent disease. So when I talk about prophylactic antibiotics in this book, I am referring to antibiotics that are given to women in the hope of preventing EOGBS disease in their baby.

You will also see the abbreviation IAP in some of the quotes in this book and in other literature on this topic. IAP stands for *intrapartum antibiotic prophylaxis*, which is a medical term used to describe the antibiotics that are offered to some women via a drip in labour. *Intrapartum* simply describes the period of labour and birth. A few other forms of prophylaxis are used and discussed in relation to GBS, and I talk about these in chapter three. There is an important difference between prophylactic antibiotics, which are offered 'just in case' and antibiotics that are offered as a treatment when someone is known to have an infection. I will discuss examples of this later.

I am going to return to defining a few other important words and terms below, but I want to first begin a conversation about language which I think is even more important than the one about jargon. Some women say that they feel dirty as a result of the language (and possibly the approach) that is used when GBS is discussed. They don't like being told that they are infected with something, or having information presented in a way that suggests they are unclean. Others dislike the term 'GBS positive' because it sounds similar to the unrelated term 'HIV positive'. It's also inaccurate because it doesn't clearly indicate that GBS bacteria can come and go. In other words, having GBS bacteria on your body at one point in time doesn't mean you've always had them there, or that you always will.

Some of this negative terminology has probably arisen because, for decades, Western culture as a whole has focused more on the kinds of bacteria that cause disease rather than presenting bacteria as organisms that can be helpful (or, as yogurt adverts like to suggest, even friendly) or just benign. This isn't necessarily something that health professionals can easily address, and I would like to hope that this might already be changing as there is now far more focus on the positive elements of bacteria as part of the human microbiome, a term that refers to all of the micro-organisms that live on and in our bodies - including, of course, happy yogurt bacteria (Turnbaugh *et al* 2007, Collado *et al* 2012).

I have already explained that GBS bacteria are, in the vast majority of cases, benign residents of the human body. When someone has a certain kind of bacteria living on or in their body, even if the bacteria are benign, they are sometimes said to be *colonised* by that bacteria. But while the biological definition of colonisation simply means that a species has moved to a particular area of the body or planet, in other contexts the term colonised is used to refer to the takeover of a place by settlers. This is why some people feel uncomfortable with that word.

If a type of bacteria is (or becomes) harmful, then terms such as *infection* or *infected* tend to be used, and these might well be appropriate when we are talking about a baby who has already become ill, but some people and texts use this term to refer to anybody who has GBS bacteria in or on their body. This can feel like even more of an invasion and it isn't necessarily appropriate language when talking about a woman who simply happens to be one of the 20 per cent (or so, depending on where you live) of people for whom GBS bacteria are a part of their microbiome on that day.

These issues were discussed by MacDonald *et al* (2010) in an analysis of texts and practices relating to GBS. They noted that GBS bacteria are often personified, or endowed with human characteristics, which *"gives the impression that GBS is an enemy and out to kill 'vulnerable' babies."* These midwives also found that many of the books and papers that discuss GBS use *"war talk ... words and phrases that might otherwise be found in the context of war and battle."* *"In the obstetric and paediatric literature, a woman has a 'colonization status' and infection statistics are 'attack rates'."* Further examples increase the idea that the bacteria acts intentionally and strategically: *"'immediate or delayed invasion of host defences' and 'the amniotic fluid is infected from the ascending vaginal route' as if part of a tactical invasion"* (MacDonald *et al* 2010: 49).

At this point in time, I am not sure that there is a good answer to the question of what language we should use. There is a need for balance, and I don't want to underplay the severity of EOGBS disease by not using terms such as infected or infection when they are appropriate (such as when talking about a baby who has EOGBS disease), but militaristic language and language that might makes people feel dirty or invaded is clearly inappropriate, so I am going to try and use everyday language – like carry, carriage or carrier – whenever possible and only use terms like colonised when I really have to, for instance because I am quoting research findings and I have to use the language of the original text in order to share with you what the authors found or said. In the longer term, it is my hope that increased discussion of these issues might help us to come up with better, more appropriate and more woman-centred language in this and many other birth-related areas.

How common is GBS carriage?

We have known for many years that the prevalence of GBS carriage varies a lot between different geographical regions (Whitney *et al* 2004), and you don't always have to travel far to see significant differences appearing. For instance, one of the first systematic reviews of studies carried out in the UK showed that 18.1% of women carry GBS overall, but there was substantial variation in the proportion of GBS carriers in different areas of the UK (Colbourn & Gilbert 2007).

Barcaite *et al* (2008) determined that the range of GBS carriage in Europe also varied, with regional carriage rates of 19.7-29.3% in Eastern Europe, 11-21% in Western Europe, 24.3-36% in Scandinavia, and 6.5-32% in Southern Europe. Since then, a number of researchers have published studies looking at the prevalence of GBS carriage in their hospitals or regions, and the variation in this becomes even more marked when we consider studies carried out in different areas of the world. It's also important to remember that these are also only 'snapshots', because GBS bacteria 'come and go'.

I have listed below the results of a few studies showing the rates of GBS carriage found in different countries at a time when this was being measured in research studies. Some of these studies are now a few years old and that is because this isn't something that is regularly monitored. The studies are also of variable quality, but I'm really just trying to illustrate the diversity of findings. In each case, I will list the location of the study and then the percentage of women who were found to carry GBS. I have added rough estimates of the likelihood as well, as this is often easier for many people to make sense of than percentages.

A snapshot of GBS carriage rates in:

Mozambique: 1.8% (1 in 55) (de Steenwinkel *et al* 2008).

Bangladesh: 7.7% (1 in 13) (Chan *et al* 2013).

Lithuania: 8.3% (1 in 12) (Barcaite *et al* 2012).

Korea: 10% (1 in 10) (Hong *et al* 2010).

Saudi Arabia: 13.4% (1 in 7) (Khan *et al* 2015).

The Netherlands: 14% (1 in 7) (Tajik *et al* 2014).

Germany: 17-18.5%, depending on test (Kunze *et al* 2015).

Lebanon: 17.7% (1 in 6) (Seoud *et al* 2010).

Italy: 18.1% (1 in 6) (Berardi *et al* 2011).

USA: 19.5% (1 in 5) (Knudtson *et al* 2010).

New Zealand: 22% (1 in 5) (Grimwood *et al* 2002).

Tanzania: 23% (1 in 4) (Joachim *et al* 2009).

Australia: 23% (1 in 4) (Garland & Kelly 1995).

Ghana: 25.5% to 28% (1 in 4) (Slotved *et al* 2017).

Zimbabwe: 60.3% (3 in 5) (Mavenyengwa *et al* 2010).

You may have spotted a few trends in that list, and a more recent systematic review analysed a whopping 221 different studies from around the world to see whether or not there were general trends. The authors found that: *"The estimated mean prevalence of rectovaginal group B streptococcus colonisation was 17·9% (95% CI 16·2–19·7) overall and was highest in Africa (22·4, 18·1–26·7) followed by the Americas (19·7, 16·7–22·7) and Europe (19·0, 16·1–22·0). Studies from southeast Asia had the lowest estimated mean prevalence (11·1%, 95% CI 6·8–15·3)"* (Kwatra et al 2016).

A few studies have considered whether there are factors that affect the likelihood that a person carries GBS. A study by Stapleton et al (2005) suggested that ethnicity, BMI (or body mass index, a measure of whether someone weighs more or less than average) and occupation may play a part. Their results showed that black women, women with a higher than average BMI and health care workers had higher rates of GBS carriage than average. Researchers in Barcelona, Spain, found that women who experienced higher ambient temperatures and humidity had a higher chance of carrying GBS (Dadvand et al 2011). It is important to understand that these studies, while very interesting, were also relatively small, and some of these findings were quite marginal. Larger studies carried out in other areas may well produce different findings.

There may be other factors that affect the likelihood that a person carries GBS. We don't know enough about how vaginal GBS carriage changes with sexual activity or factors such as condom use, although there is evidence that GBS colonisation may be more likely if a woman has a new sex partner, multiple sex partners or frequent sex (Foxman et al 2007). Research has also shown that GBS can be passed back and forth during partner-to-woman oral sex (Foxman et al 2008). We don't know whether having candida (thrush) or a bacterial infection in the vagina has an effect on GBS. We don't know whether GBS has a role in our bodies that we don't yet understand, or whether it doesn't really belong in the vagina and it only appears because something is out of balance with the person's microbiome. It might be affected by what a person eats, by other environmental factors, or by the state of her immune system. There are many things we have yet to discover.

There is no way of knowing whether you are carrying GBS or not unless you have a test to find out. As I have mentioned, GBS is not something that people 'get' and have forever. It is possible for a person to be found to be carrying GBS one week and not the next, and vice versa. But we don't know how much of this is because GBS bacteria 'come and go' or because the tests aren't as sensitive as they might be. This is quite an important consideration when we come (in chapter two) to look at the timing and accuracy of screening tests for women who choose to have these.

So how do you know if you carry GBS?

The usual way of determining that a woman is carrying GBS is for a laboratory to analyse a swab of her vagina and rectum (back passage) or perianal area, which is the area around the anus. The rectum or perianal area is almost always swabbed as well as the vagina because studies have shown that taking a vaginal swab alone is not as effective at detecting GBS carriage. It is also thought that bacteria can be present in the rectal or perianal area but absent from the vagina and yet still transferred to the baby at birth. Colbourn and Gilbert's (2007) review, for instance, found that 14% of women were found to be carrying GBS when vaginal swabs are used, but this rose to the 18.1% quoted above when swabs of their rectal area were tested as well. However, I haven't found any data on the rates of EOGBS disease in relation to where a positive test was obtained from. Research has shown that it is as effective to swab the perianal area as inside the anus, and less unpleasant for women, who may find it uncomfortable and embarrassing to have a swab inserted into their anus (Jamie *et al* 2004, Trappe *et al* 2011).

GBS can also sometimes be detected when a urine sample is tested for bacteria, and there are some important things to know about this. Research has suggested that women who have GBS bacteria in their urine have a higher chance of having an affected baby (Schrag *et al* 2002) and national guidelines often suggest that a finding of GBS in the urine should mean that a woman is offered antibiotics in labour (Darlow *et al* 2015, Hughes *et al* 2017). However, in some countries, including the UK, urine testing alone isn't usually used to test for GBS and we would only usually find out that GBS was present in a woman's urine if she had a urine test for other reasons. In the past, the kind of urine testing that would discover GBS (that is, when a urine sample is put into a pot and tested at a laboratory; GBS can't be found using the 'dipstick' test that midwives and doctors use) was usually only carried out when a woman had symptoms suggestive of a urinary tract infection. More recently, however, I have learned that some areas are offering routine urine testing in early pregnancy. This is worrying, because women are being given a sample pot by someone who is not a health professional (for example a receptionist at a doctor's surgery) and asked to urinate in it without being told that they are being screened for possible GBS and that the results may significantly affect their care and the options that they will be offered. We will return to this issue later in the book.

A GBS swab test shouldn't be painful, but if it is carried out by a health professional then the woman will need to undress and lie on her back with her legs apart, a position which some women find embarrassing or uncomfortable, especially in late pregnancy or labour. The swabs are like long cotton buds and, if the test is performed by a midwife or doctor, she or he will insert the swab just inside the vagina, gently rotate it and then withdraw it. The midwife or doctor will then insert another swab into the anus, rotate it and remove it or touch the swab to the outside of the anus, rotate it and remove it. Because of the risk of introducing harmful bacteria into the vagina, the vagina should always be swabbed before the rectum or perianal area. A different swab should be used for each.

Instead of doing the test themselves, some midwives and doctors will ask the woman if she would prefer to take a swab to a bathroom and perform the test herself. Like inserting a tampon or menstrual cup, this can be done in one of a number of positions, according to personal preference. If you decide to undergo GBS testing but do not like the thought of someone else carrying it out, you can tell your care provider that you wish to do the swabbing yourself. The swab is then placed in a tube which is labelled and sent to a laboratory for analysis.

Women who have symptoms of vaginal infection, such as itching, discomfort or an unusual or smelly discharge, are offered a similar test in which a swab is used to take a sample from the upper or lower vagina. The swab can then be tested for a number of different kinds of bacteria, which may include GBS. Although it is not considered to be a common cause of vaginal infection, GBS is sometimes picked up on such a test. This is why, as I will discuss in more depth later, women need to be aware of the implications of having a swab test during pregnancy, as well as any urine test (other than the 'dipstick' testing, as I explained above). More information on the types, timing and funding of testing can be found in chapter two of this book. I should note, however, that GBS testing is not routinely recommended in countries such as the UK and New Zealand, because a different approach to determining risk is used.

Neonatal GBS disease

We have already established that GBS is a bacterium which a percentage of people carry in their bodies and that, while we don't think it offers any particular advantage to the carrier, it is usually not considered harmful or unhealthy. I have also explained that GBS can exist in the vagina or rectum (among other places) and so, when a woman who carries GBS becomes pregnant and gives birth, the GBS bacteria can sometimes be transferred to her baby during labour and birth. Most of the time this is not a problem, and every day thousands of women with GBS in their vaginas and/or rectums give birth to healthy babies. When we collect swabs from the skin of babies born to women who are known to have the GBS bacteria in their vagina, we find that about half of these babies have picked up GBS during their birth, and about half haven't. Although most of the babies who carry GBS bacteria are healthy and well, every now and then a baby who picks up the GBS bacteria around the time of birth becomes very ill.

What we don't know, as I will discuss here, is whether all of the babies who develop EOGBS disease are getting the GBS bacteria from their mothers, or whether some of those bacteria are being transferred by other family members or health professionals. The assumption has been that GBS is only transmitted from woman to baby, especially when the disease appears early, but this is worth questioning.

GBS disease in newly born babies is said to occur in two time frames.

Early onset GBS (EOGBS) disease is the one we are focusing on in this book. It occurs during the first seven days of life, although 90 per cent of cases begin within the first 24 hours of life. It is more likely to occur in babies who are born prematurely, who are small, whose mothers' waters released more than 12 hours before they gave birth or who have one or more of a number of other risk factors (Ohlsson & Shah 2014, Yagupsky *et al* 1991). It is almost (but not quite) exclusively seen in babies born to women who already carry GBS bacteria. When bacteria are transmitted from a mother to a baby, the term *vertical transmission* may be used.

There is a general belief that, at this early stage, there are not many ways for a baby to pick up the bacteria other than from its mother, but babies are often handled by health care workers who may carry GBS on their hands. They may also encounter equipment or furniture with GBS bacteria on it.

This is not something that has been discussed a lot in the literature. In fact, Ohlsson & Shah (2014) propose that, in the few cases where babies have been born to women who had negative GBS test results, there may have been false negative results or other test-related errors.

There is a long history of medical professionals being unable to imagine that they themselves may be the cause of diseases or problems, so we should not be too surprised by the lack of research into this area. A recent exception to this has arisen in the form of a study by Åberg *et al* (2018) which discussed how GBS bacteria had affected a number of babies in a neonatal unit. GBS was found on surfaces near the sick and colonised babies and it is likely to have been transferred via equipment and staff.

Early symptoms of EOGBS disease include fever (a high temperature), feeding difficulties, making grunting noises, irritability, lethargy (being limp or hard to wake), breathing difficulties, unusual heart rate and/or a blue-ish tinge to the skin (which is less easy to spot in darker-skinned babies). Not all babies with GBS disease will have all of these symptoms, and many babies who have one or more of these symptoms don't have EOGBS disease.

GBS disease can develop very quickly. A baby with EOGBS disease may develop septicaemia (infection of the blood), pneumonia (inflammation of the lungs) and/or meningitis (inflammation of the brain and spinal cord). A baby who is thought to be affected by GBS disease will be commenced on treatment as soon as possible, with that treatment including antibiotics which are usually given intravenously.

Late onset GBS disease is the term used to describe GBS disease when it occurs between seven days and up to three months of age. Factors that increase the chance of a baby developing late onset GBS disease include non-white race and preterm birth (Yagupsky *et al* 1991). Late onset GBS disease is not usually associated with pregnancy and the

18

baby is likely to have encountered the GBS bacteria after birth. In contrast to the vertical transmission of EOGBS disease, late onset GBS disease is said to be spread by *horizontal transmission* (Morinis *et al* 2011). Late onset GBS disease is not preventable by any intervention that we can offer during pregnancy or labour, and we will not be looking further at this in this book.

Putting the risk into context

The incidence and outcomes of EOGBS disease varies according to time, place and perhaps the measures being taken to reduce it. This point is illustrated well by looking at recent changes in our understanding of the risks for babies.

The first question that we need to ask here is how many babies would be affected by EOGBS disease if we did nothing, and an answer to this is provided by Homer *et al* (2014), whose analysis showed that, *"...without prophylactic intervention, the incidence of EOGBSD in Australia, the United States and Western Europe has been estimated at between 0.4 and 4 per 1000 live births."* That is between 1 in 250 and 1 in 2500 babies. In 2013, the UK figure was 1 in 2000 babies, and the Royal College of Obstetricians and Gynaecologists (RGOC) guideline which was current at that time summarised what this meant for those babies:

"One in every 2000 newborn babies in the UK and Ireland is diagnosed with GBS infection. Although the infection can make the baby very unwell, with prompt treatment the majority (7 out of 10 of diagnosed babies) recover fully. However, 2 in 10 babies with GBS infection will recover with some level of disability, and 1 in 10 infected babies will die. Overall, 1 in 17 000 newborn babies in the UK and Ireland die from the infection" (RCOG 2013: 1).

But knowledge moves on with time, and the data used by the RCOG in the previous paragraph are based upon surveillance data gathered and analysed in the year 2000. A more recent surveillance report (O'Sullivan *et al* 2019) showed that the incidence of EOGBS disease in the UK had risen (from 0.48 in 1000 babies in the year 2000 to 0.57 in 1000 babies in 2015), but it also showed that the risk of death from EOGBS disease had gone down, from 10.6% to 5.2%. So from those data, we can say that 1 in 1750 babies born in the UK will be diagnosed with EOGBS disease, and the chance of death from EOGBS disease in the UK is 1 in 33,738. This study also showed that 7.4% of babies with EOGBS disease will recover but have an ongoing health issue, a figure which is slightly lower than in the data gathered in 2000. Data from similar surveillance carried out in New Zealand have shown that the rate of EOGBS disease has halved in the ten years between surveys (Darlow *et al* 2015).

Another very helpful set of figures was shared by Bevan *et al* (2019) who undertook a mapping exercise "...*to estimate the potential impact of the addition of culture-based screening for group B streptococcus (GBS) carriage in pregnancy to a risk-based prevention policy in the UK.*" Bevan *et al* (2019) calculated the number of women who would need to be given intravenous antibiotics in labour to prevent each case of EOGBS disease. They showed that, with the current risk-based programme, "*30,666 women were estimated to receive IAP and 70 cases of EOGBS were prevented.*" When we account for the fact that between 89.4% and 96% of babies survive EOGBS disease (Bevan *et al* 2019), we can see that, under the current risk-based programme, we would need to give intravenous antibiotics to around 2190 women in labour to prevent one case of death or serious morbidity from EOGBS disease.

But not all babies are equally at risk from EOGBS disease and before we move on to look at Bevan *et al*'s (2019) calculations for universal GBS screening, it is important to know that some babies are more likely to be affected by EOGBS disease than others. This is another key reason why some countries use a risk-based screening approach, which I will discuss in chapter two. O'Sullivan *et al*'s (2019) research showed that 22% of the babies who developed GBS disease had been born prematurely. We know that the mortality (death) risk from EOGBS disease is very different in babies born at full term and babies who are born preterm. The US-based Centers for Disease Control and Prevention (CDC 2010a) showed that preterm babies are at greater risk than babies born at term if they develop EOGBS disease. The mortality rate of those babies who were born at 33 weeks gestation or earlier is 20-30 per cent (so between 1 in 3 and 1 in 5). The survival rate from EOGBS disease increases with gestational age and babies born at full term (that is, after 37 or more completed weeks of pregnancy) have a far lower chance of dying if they have EOGBS disease, at 2-3% (or between 1 in 33 and 1 in 50). In other words, the mortality risk from EOGBS disease is ten times higher in preterm babies than in babies born at full term (after 37 weeks of pregnancy).

So the level of risk is very different depending on when a woman goes into labour. Women who are 37 or more weeks pregnant when they go into labour may find it useful to know that Bevan *et al*'s (2019) mapping showed that *"The likelihood of having a baby affected by EOGBS appears to be low in women delivering at term with no known risk factors; a rate of about 0.2/1,000 live births was used in the model."* In other words, the unborn baby of a healthy woman who goes into labour at term and who does not have other risk factors (which we will look at more in chapter two), has a 1 in 5000 chance of being affected by EOGBS and a 1 in 39,682 chance of experiencing death or serious illness following EOGBS.

When we look at those figures, it becomes clearer why some countries are not moving towards a universal, culture-based screening programme and instead focus on babies who are at particular risk. It is also easy to understand why some women decide to avoid screening or prophylaxis altogether. In the absence of risk factors, the chance of an adverse outcome from EOGBS disease is incredibly low. Even where risk factors exist, the chance is still very low, but it is of course up to each woman to decide what is right for her and her baby.

Bevan *et al* (2019) also looked at the impact of universal, culture-based screening on the number of women who would be offered antibiotics in labour as well as on the outcomes for babies. They found that, theoretically, if the UK adopted a universal GBS screening programme, we might be able to prevent three EOGBS deaths and four cases of severe disability each year. However, an additional 96,260 women would be offered intravenous antibiotics in labour each year. That would mean up to 126,926 women having intravenous antibiotics in labour as GBS prophylaxis every year, which is 17.8% of all women in labour. This figure doesn't include women who would be offered antibiotics for other reasons. It does include between 16,382 and 24,065 women who would be offered antibiotics because they had been carrying GBS at the time of testing but who would no longer be carrying GBS by the time they gave birth (Bevan *et al* 2019).

It is really important to look at the wider picture of what we do and do not know in this area. As the above figures show, although pressure groups are stressing the increase in diagnosed cases of EOGBS disease, advances in the care and treatment of sick babies mean that fewer babies are dying and having long-term problems as a result of EOGBS disease. There are also, as we will consider later in the book, risks to screening and prophylaxis, and there is a need to weigh up the pros and cons of each possible course of action.

Summarising the dilemmas

As the figures in the previous section show, EOGBS disease can be deadly, but it is rare. Improved sanitation and living standards and advances in health care have reduced the risk of infectious disease dramatically but this has also changed the balance so that previously rare conditions (such as EOGBS disease) that are hard to completely eradicate are now seen as the biggest problems that we need to solve. EOGBS disease is now the most common cause of infection in newborns born at full term (Vergnano *et al* 2010, Stoll 2011, Hughes *et al* 2017). (The most common cause of infection in preterm babies is caused by the *E. coli* bacteria.) But some people find the use of the word 'common' in that statement to be a bit confusing when they look at the actual numbers.

Because EOGBS disease can be fatal, it is easy to understand why the focus on screening and offering prophylaxis for GBS has increased in recent years. But the actions that are taken to screen for and treat GBS carriage carry risks in themselves. So we have a complex situation with several different facets to take into consideration and no one right answer. Instead, there is a lot of disagreement about whether we should offer screening and preventative measures to women with regard to GBS and, if so, what form these should take.

The first guidelines relating to the prevention of EOGBS disease were published in the US (AAP 1992, ACOG 1992) and the first UK guideline was published by the RCOG in 2003 (Hughes *et al* 2003). But these guidelines and the versions that have followed them are very different from each other, because of differences in opinion. Broadly, two very different approaches are taken. Parts of the US, Australia and several European countries take one approach, and other countries, such as the UK and New Zealand, take another. Chapter two of this book looks at the different approaches to determining which babies are deemed to be at risk from EOGBS disease.

2. Screening, testing and risk

There has been a movement in health care over the past few decades towards trying to identify people who are at high risk of having a certain problem or disease. If we know that a person is at risk of something, an attempt can be made to either prevent it, minimise the risk or treat it in the early stages before it becomes serious. Such is the basis for recommendations about breast self-examination, regular check-ups for people who have diabetes and the questionnaires administered to people in hospitals and care homes to determine who is at risk of getting bedsores. In this chapter, I will look at the evidence and recommendations that relate to whether and how we should try and determine which babies are at risk from EOGBS disease.

Explaining screening

Pregnant women are offered more screening tests than any other group of healthy people. Most of the things that midwives and doctors do during pregnancy are screening tests. We check women's blood pressure and urine and palpate women's abdomens to see if their uterus and baby are the 'right' size, the 'right' way up and in the 'right' position, and this is only in the first five minutes of the antenatal appointment. All of these activities are screening tests and, if the results of any of these measurements are not within normal limits, clinicians may recommend some kind of action as a result. Depending on whether the screening test is looking for an actual problem or a sign that someone is at risk of a problem, the recommended action might be actual treatment, more screening or check-ups or some kind of preventative (or prophylactic) measure.

So when clinicians first decided they needed to address the problem of EOGBS disease, it was perhaps inevitable that their first step would be to search for an effective way to screen for the problem. It is very important to remember, however, that screening is only useful if we also have an effective form of prevention or treatment to offer to those babies who are deemed to be at risk of a problem. I'll look at the question of prophylactic approaches for the prevention of EOGBS disease in chapter three of this book.

Two very different approaches to GBS-related screening emerged, and both remain quite crude. In a few regions, a combination of the two approaches is used, but most areas of the world have picked either one or the other.

Before we look at these two approaches to GBS-related screening in detail, I'd like to explain a bit about what we're looking for when we create a screening test such as the one used to identify whether or not a woman is carrying GBS bacteria. It is my hope that this will help you to better understand the pros and cons of the current approaches. For instance, as you will see in the list below, a good screening test will identify as many of the people who have a particular problem as possible, while not identifying too many people as being 'at risk' if they don't have the problem. These elements are referred to as sensitivity and specificity, which I will explain further below. These elements relate to both approaches to GBS-related screening but in this example I am going to focus on the screening test that looks at whether a woman is carrying GBS bacteria.

As I also explain throughout this book, neither of the current approaches to screening for GBS disease are particularly sensitive or specific, and this has repercussions for women and babies. A lack of sensitivity means that, even though many women are offered antibiotics in labour with both approaches, a proportion of babies will still develop EOGBS disease. Low specificity leads to overtreatment.

Some of the important factors against which we can measure a screening test include:

26

Sensitivity, or how good the test is at picking up a disease (or, in this case, a certain kind of bacteria) when it is present. Poor sensitivity leads to a high false negative rate, which in the case of GBS would describe the situation where a woman is carrying GBS bacteria but this is not picked up by the screening test. She would be told that she didn't have the bacteria and thus she would not be offered antibiotics.

Specificity, which is how good a test is at *only* identifying people who have the bacteria. Poor specificity leads to a higher false positive rate which leads to more women who do not have the bacteria being told they are carrying it and being offered unnecessary antibiotics. This is a big concern with GBS screening, especially in countries where universal bacteriological (culture-based) screening is used.

Practical considerations: whether the test can be carried out with the facilities and staff available (for instance, tests requiring electrical equipment are not feasible in some countries or locations).

Staffing considerations: who can carry out the test, and whether they need to be specially trained. Currently, the tests are carried out in a laboratory but there are moves towards screening that can be carried out on labour wards. I will discuss this further below.

Speed of testing: how long it takes to get a result.

Cost: some laboratory tests are expensive, and this can make a difference to whether it is feasible to offer the test given the available budget and priorities.

Acceptability of screening method: whether women are OK with how the sample is collected, tested and the result reported to them.

Each of these has to be balanced against the others, and in reality most tests in any area of midwifery or medicine have advantages and disadvantages. One last thing to mention before I discuss the specific types of test that are used in an attempt to detect GBS is that, although the term 'gold standard' is sometimes used to describe the test that is currently considered the best, we cannot be certain that any test is one hundred per cent effective at determining whether or not bacteria are present. Because how do we know, and what are we measuring these tests against?

In theory, we can do research and find that test X picks up more cases than test Y, but although that might be because test X is more sensitive and better at detecting the bacteria than test Y, it might instead be that test X has a high false positive rate. I mention this because all of these tests can only be measured against each other and it is important to remember that, while science, medicine and technology are great tools in our quest for knowledge, they are by no means infallible.

Culture-based and risk-based screening

One approach to screening for EOGBS disease is to offer all pregnant women a test in late pregnancy to see if they have GBS bacteria in or around their vagina or rectum. This is the approach currently taken in much of the US, many parts of Canada and Australia and several European countries, including Spain, Belgium and Finland. This approach is called universal, bacteriological or culture-based screening.

If the test shows that the woman is carrying GBS bacteria, she will be offered intravenous antibiotics during labour. As we saw in chapter one, when I listed the percentages of people who have been found to carry GBS in studies undertaken in different countries and regions, this means that, on average, somewhere between a fifth to a quarter of all pregnant women are offered intravenous antibiotics in labour. Some people consider this to be a significant level of overtreatment, but proponents of this approach see it as the best way to offer protection to as many babies as possible. Other countries, such as the UK and New Zealand, take a different approach. Rather than routinely offering laboratory testing for GBS and then offering antibiotics in labour to all of the 20-25% of women who are found to be carrying the bacteria at the time of testing, antibiotics are offered to women in labour whose babies are deemed to be at higher risk of getting an infection if their mothers are carrying GBS. This includes women/babies who have certain risk factors, such as being in preterm labour. A good many women are still offered antibiotics where risk-based screening is used, but not quite as many as with culture-based screening. We will look at specific risk factors in much more detail below.

In both the UK and New Zealand, the decision to recommend risk-based screening was a deliberate one, based on concerns about the overtreatment that results from culture-based screening. In the UK, the National Screening Committee (2008, 2017) has maintained the position that it does not recommend routine bacteriological testing for GBS carriage in the antenatal period. This position has, if anything, been strengthened by more recent work by O'Sullivan *et al* (2019) and Bevan *et al* (2019) and the RCOG states that universal screening will not be considered, *'until it is clear that antenatal screening for GBS carriage does more good than harm and that the benefits are cost-effective'* (2013: 3). I discussed the data that relate to this in chapter one.

The most recent RCOG Green-top guideline (Hughes *et al* 2017) quotes the National Screening Committee's position, offering further insight into the reasons for this decision and the arguments against universal bacteriological screening:

"The National Screening Committee does not recommend universal bacteriological screening for GBS. Their view is that there is no clear evidence to show that testing for GBS routinely would do more good than harm. The reasons quoted are:

Many women carry the bacteria and, in the majority of cases, their babies are born safely and without developing an infection. Screening women late in pregnancy cannot accurately predict which babies will develop GBS infection.

No screening test is entirely accurate. Between 17% and 25% of women who have a positive swab at 35–37 weeks of gestation will be GBS negative at delivery. Between 5% and 7% of women who are GBS negative at 35–37 weeks of gestation will be GBS positive at delivery.

In addition, many of the babies who are severely affected from GBS infection are born prematurely, before the suggested time for screening.

Giving all carriers of GBS IAP would mean that a very large number of women would receive treatment they do not need; this may increase adverse outcomes to mother and baby" (Hughes et al 2017: e289).

Further support for this position came in early 2019, when Seedat et al (2019) published an analysis of this issue in the British Medical Journal. Among other things, they noted that, "The current approach to screening would lead to 99.8% of screen positive women and their babies receiving unnecessary intrapartum antibiotic prophylaxis" (Seedat et al 2019) and that, "Lack of high quality evidence on clinical outcomes makes it impossible to quantify whether universal GBS screening would have any benefit and assess whether large scale intrapartum antibiotic prophylaxis is safe" (Seedat et al 2019).

The New Zealand guideline gives similar reasons for not adopting the universal screening approach:

"The group noted that the most recent recommendation from North America was for universal screening, whilst that from the UK was for a risk-based approach. Neither will prevent all cases of EOGBS and factors such as the practicalities and cost-effectiveness need to be considered. ... A recent study (Lin et al 2011) has shown that 10% of women with negative screening were actually positive for GBS when in labour, whilst 50% of women with a positive screen result were negative for GBS when in labour. The screening approach is more expensive and exposes more women to antibiotics than the risk-based approach." (Darlow et al 2015).

Mixing the approaches

In a very few areas of the world, practitioners use a combination of these two types of screening. That is, they identify babies who have risk factors, and then offer their mothers bacteriological screening. This can help reduce the number of women and babies who receive antibiotics, as the only women who will be offered antibiotics for GBS prevention in labour are those who carry GBS *and* whose babies are deemed to be at greater risk. Antibiotics are offered to women in labour for other reasons as well as EOGBS disease prevention, of course.

It is also important to know that, even where a risk-based approach is taken, some women will still end up having a bacteriological test for GBS. A few women decide to undergo private testing for GBS. During her antenatal care, a woman might give a urine sample or have a vaginal swab taken to investigate symptoms of possible infection. In both of these situations, some of the women will be found to carry GBS and may be offered antibiotics in labour, depending on local guidelines.

In some areas where risk-based screening has been adopted, such as the UK, women who are coincidentally found to be carrying GBS will be offered antibiotics when they go into labour, even if they do not have risk factors (Hughes *et al* 2017). They may also be offered oral antibiotics during pregnancy if the GBS was found in their urine, although antibiotics will not usually be offered in pregnancy if GBS was found on a vaginal swab. But in other countries such as New Zealand (Darlow *et al* 2015), women who are found to be carrying GBS in early pregnancy will be offered further testing later in pregnancy. This is because, as above, we know that the GBS bacteria may not be present when the woman goes into labour, and offering testing again in late pregnancy helps reduce the number of women who are offered antibiotics.

Women may also be offered antibiotics in pregnancy or labour if they have signs of an infection. Signs of infection in a woman before or during labour might include a raised temperature and/or pulse, uterine (womb) tenderness and/or an unusual vaginal discharge. In this situation, the main concern is to protect the woman and the kind of antibiotic that is offered may or may not be the same kind that would be offered to try to protect the baby from EOGBS disease. Again, it depends on local guidelines.

Which approach is best?

There is a lot of debate amongst women, midwives, doctors and birth workers about which of these approaches is best and whether it would be better to take a completely different approach or not screen at all. As much of this book will show, all of the approaches in current use have significant downsides, mostly in relation to overtreatment, the consequences of giving so many antibiotics and the restriction of women's options. But they are understandable responses to the problem. Homer *et al* (2014) carried out an analysis of the existing international guidelines and concluded that both culture-based and risk-based approaches to the prevention of EOGBS could be recommended as reasonable from a medical perspective given the state of our knowledge of this area. They concluded that the standard of the guidelines in most countries was high and that there was a lack of clear evidence showing that either approach was better than the other. This lack of clear evidence is an ongoing problem.

Individual women and practitioners may agree or disagree with the approach offered in their region, as the differences very much relate to overall beliefs about birth, health and risk. Some women living in areas such as the UK and New Zealand that use risk-based screening choose to pay for a private bacteriological GBS test. Other women are very happy that these countries have resisted adopting an approach that would lead to even more women being offered antibiotics in labour and further restrict some women from being able to make the decisions that are right for them. I hear from a lot of women in Australia, Europe and the USA who feel they do not want screening (but, in many cases, do not know how to resist it), while many others do not question the recommendations, assuming that health professionals or policymakers must know best.

Another important factor is that there are also some significant differences in midwifery and obstetric practice around the world and between different practitioners in the same country. Women giving birth in maternity care systems in the US and Australia will, on the whole, experience more medicalised maternity care than women giving birth in countries such as New Zealand and the UK. They are likely to experience more vaginal examinations (including during pregnancy in the USA) and other interventions which may affect the number of babies who develop EOGBS disease.

A small study by Knudtson *et al* (2010) suggested that vaginal examination in late pregnancy didn't make a huge difference to whether a woman tests positive for GBS and, if anything, the likelihood of testing positive for GBS is reduced immediately afterwards, but this study had a number of limitations and only looked at the results of a GBS test immediately following the vaginal examination. Given the concerns that I noted in chapter one about whether GBS could be transmitted by health professionals and equipment during birth, it would also be useful to know whether and how birth interventions in labour and the early postnatal period made a difference to the number of babies who develop EOGBS disease.

In many areas of the US and some other countries which take a universal culture-based screening approach, women routinely have intravenous drips in labour, and this may arguably make intravenous antibiotics seem like less of an additional intrusion in labour, although it will depend very much on the feelings of the individual woman. There are also other differences in intervention rates between countries, and the caesarean section rate in these more medicalised countries is also higher than in many of the countries using risk-based screening, including the UK and New Zealand. For all of these reasons, caution should be used when making comparisons between policies and outcomes in countries which have such different approaches to maternity care. The RCOG (2012) reached the same conclusion and considered that "extrapolation of practice from the USA to the UK may ... be inappropriate" (2).

Because EOGBS disease is rare and the risks of antibiotics are significant, some women choose not to have any testing in pregnancy that might detect GBS unless they feel this is truly necessary for a different problem. This is to avoid being urged to take antibiotics for EOGBS disease prevention, and in some cases because having a positive GBS test result may restrict a woman's options, for instance where women are told that they are not able to give birth in a birth centre, a midwifery led unit or at home if they are known to be carrying GBS. While a woman cannot legally be stopped from giving birth at home, I know of cases where women have been declined entry to a midwifery-led birth centre and this situation has led to significant distress.

Culture-based screening for GBS

I have already shared some of the downsides of culture-based screening from the perspective of authorities in the UK (Hughes *et al* 2017) and New Zealand (Darlow *et al* 2015). So what reason do countries such as the US and Australia have for using this approach?

The answer to this question is complex. It is partly due to the modern trend wherein we have a tendency to focus on doing everything possible to prevent potential problems, even if there isn't any evidence that the things that we are doing are effective. This tendency has arisen in the past few decades and social scientists have helped us understand that the approach taken to childbirth is not always logical or evidence-based and that there are a number of different perspectives that people can take towards life and birth in general and in relation to these sorts of decisions (Oakley 1980, 1984, Davis-Floyd 1992, Murphy-Lawless 1998, Edwards 2005, Wickham 2018a). I have written about these approaches in my book, *"What's Right For Me: making decisions in pregnancy and childbirth"* (Wickham 2018a).

The evidence usually cited in support of universal, culture-based screening is that EOGBS disease rates have significantly improved since this kind of screening was implemented. For instance, a CDC (2010a) report shows that EOGBS disease rates have dropped from 1.7 cases per 1,000 births in the early 1990s to 0.25 cases per 1,000 births when the report was published. However, as I discussed in the previous section, we cannot be certain that this is due to the screening and prophylaxis methods being used. There are other possible reasons for this change, and we have also seen changes in EOGBS disease rates in countries using risk-based screening. There is also, as I will explain in the next section, a lack of evidence from randomised controlled trials to show that giving antibiotics is effective.

As we have seen, universal, culture-based screening leads to an overuse of antibiotics but it does not identify every woman who is carrying GBS bacteria. We also know from Bienenfeld *et al* (2016) that it is hard to implement this approach. In their research, carried out in the USA, about 40% of women who were known to carry GBS when tested during pregnancy did not receive the recommended dose of antibiotics when they were in labour. In the majority of cases this was unavoidable, not because the antibiotics were forgotten, but because birth occurred before enough time had passed for them to be effective or for another reason that nobody could help or change. Another study, this time carried out in Italy, came up with similar results. About half of eligible women weren't offered screening and about half of those who were found to be carrying GBS didn't receive antibiotics in labour (de Luca *et al* 2015).

The authors of the Italian study felt that some things could be done to improve these rates, but I want to return to the American study, whose authors found that the majority of situations where the protocol wasn't followed were unavoidable. As we will see later, there is a large question mark over whether antibiotics are effective in preventing EOGBS disease. But even if they are effective when given at the right dose, the fact that 40% of the women who are being given them are being given a less then optimal dose is a serious issue to consider, and it is inextricably linked to the question of whether the different screening approaches are effective and ethical.

Women are often advised to go to hospital early if they are going to have antibiotics for EOGBS disease prevention, and this is so that they can have had at least four hours' worth of antibiotics before the baby is born. It is thought that this dose and timeframe is the most effective. But women who are likely to have a short labour (for instance because they have a history of this, or because they have had several babies before) are not usually advised to consider their antibiotic decision in the light of this. On the other hand, proponents of intravenous antibiotics claim that, although at least four hours' worth of coverage with benzyl penicillin is optimal, having antibiotics for any length of time is better than nothing and will confer some protection to the baby. The existence of these many viewpoints and complex debates shows why some prefer an approach more geared to the individual woman and her baby.

Some of these issues will be better understood if I explain exactly what happens when bacteriological screening is carried out, so let's look at that next. The issues that I am about to discuss are the same no matter whether they relate to a woman who lives in a country which offers universal

36

bacteriological screening, or to a woman who lives in a country which offers risk-based screening but who has a swab test either privately or because their midwife or doctor is investigating symptoms of vaginal discharge, irritation, bleeding or possible urinary tract infection.

What happens in culture-based screening?

I described the process of swabbing the vaginal and perianal area for bacteria in chapter one. I also described how GBS bacteria may be found when urine testing is carried out, although urine testing alone is not used as a way of screening for GBS bacteria. But let's look at what happens when those swabs or samples are then sent to a laboratory for testing, as this can help explain some of the issues that exist in relation to GBS testing decisions.

Types of test for GBS

There are basically three different types of test for GBS. These are known as the direct plating method (not usually abbreviated), enriched culture medium (ECM) and polymerase chain reaction (PCR) testing. The first two of these tests are also known as culture-based tests, because they involve trying to culture or grow bacteria on a plate on which the swab has been wiped, while PCR testing uses biochemical reactions to identify whether the cells on the swab contain DNA regions that are unique to GBS bacteria. Each of these tests has advantages and disadvantages.

The **direct plating method** was the first form of testing used for GBS bacteria, and is used throughout the UK and many other countries. This kind of test is commonly carried out when a swab is taken and a midwife or doctor sends it to a pathology laboratory to see what bacteria are present in the area that was swabbed. This kind of testing wasn't created specifically to test for GBS, which is one reason that it's not the most accurate test for GBS. It was created to look for bacteria generally, for instance when a woman is thought to have a possible infection.

When the swab arrives in the laboratory, the laboratory scientist will wipe the swab or sample over a special plate (which you might also know as a petri dish) containing substances that will encourage bacteria to grow or behave in certain ways. Most culture-based tests use plates which are covered in animal (usually sheep) blood to see where certain kinds of bacteria are forming colonies (because they will haemolyse or break down blood – which is why GBS is sometimes called Beta haemolytic strep) and then these colonies are tested with chemicals to see if they contain *Streptococcus agalactiae* bacteria. Most culture-based tests need to be cultured for 48 hours before a result is available, so the results may not be ready until two or three days after the swab was taken. So this kind of test is not much help if a fast answer is needed.

Key advantages of the traditional direct plating test are that it is relatively cheap and very specific, which means that most of the women identified as carrying GBS via this test actually do carry it. However, studies comparing it with the use of a test involving an enriched culture medium (which I will discuss next) showed that it had low sensitivity. This means that it failed to pick up quite a few women who were shown as carrying GBS (Nguyen *et al* 1998). The reason for this, and the main problem with the direct plating method, is that other kinds of bacteria can also grow on the plate and mask the existence of GBS (Larsen & Sever 2008).

In many hospitals in the UK, direct plating is used to test for GBS. However, the accuracy of this test can be enhanced by use of an **enriched culture medium** (ECM). This involves adding a special broth to the plate, which will specifically encourage the growth of GBS but not other kinds of bacteria.

This increases the sensitivity of the test and ensures that more of the women who carry GBS are identified.

Again though, the results take two to three days to be available. Some people have tried to make this faster. For example, Faro *et al* (2013) found a way to accelerate culture-based testing, reducing the swab-to-result time to 6.5 hours with comparable accuracy to the existing test, but concluded that this method had disadvantages and was still unlikely to be fast enough to use when women are in labour.

The cost of ECM testing is also higher than the direct plating method, and another disadvantage is that this test can only look for GBS. This might sound like a rather obvious thing to say, but it is important to remember that the type of test carried out is determined by what the midwife or doctor is looking for.

If a midwife wants to see what bacteria are growing in general, for instance because a woman has symptoms of possible vaginal infection, then a GBS-specific medium isn't useful. That's because GBS is only one possible cause of infection and we already know that GBS infection is rarely a problem in adults. Cost, space and time are important factors, and laboratories can't set out lots of different plates, each looking for a different kind of bacteria for each woman. Consequently, traditional direct plating, which will identify the bacteria that are present, tends to be used in this situation.

If however, the test is being carried out specifically to look for GBS, then the use of a GBS-specific ECM is preferable and this is currently considered to be the best test by microbiologists. In countries (such as the UK), where routine GBS testing is not recommended, ECM testing for GBS may not be available from every hospital or laboratory.

The third kind of testing is completely different and known as **polymerase chain reaction** or PCR testing. Rather than being cultured on a plate over a couple of days, the swabs or samples are placed in a machine which uses biochemical reactions and heat to identify whether or not the cells on the swab or in the sample contain GBS-related DNA. PCR testing is not in use in the UK at the time of writing but in some areas it has been found to be more accurate, rapid and practical as an alternative to culture-based testing (Håkansson & Källén 2006, Money *et al* 2008, Daniels *et al* 2009, Abdelazim 2013, Chan *et al* 2014, Mueller *et al* 2014a). One barrier is the cost of the equipment needed to undertake PCR testing. In an analysis carried out in Saint-Étienne, France, the PCR test was found to be "prohibitively expensive" compared to culture-based testing (Poncelot-Jasserand *et al* 2013), although a team led by El Helali *et al* (2012) in Paris had calculated this to be cost-neutral in their system. This is not entirely surprising; the cost difference is likely to vary between areas, depending on issues such as the GBS carriage rate, current facilities, staffing levels and the kind of care and interventions that are offered in different circumstances. Economic evaluations of PCR testing within a UK context have led to a decision that, *"…based on their current sensitivity, specificity and cost, screening using rapid tests was dominated by other more cost-effective strategies"* (Kaambwa *et al* 2010).

Some studies have shown that sensitivity and specificity rates are similar between swabs analysed with ECM and via PCR but, when PCR testing was carried out at the point of care (that is, on the labour ward), more of the samples analysed on the labour ward are likely to be classed as invalid (Håkansson *et al* 2014, Mueller *et al* 2014a, Virranniemi *et al* 2018). This means that they have to be taken and tested again. The invalid sample rate was slightly improved by staff training (Mueller *et al* 2014a), but labour ward staff are less experienced at sample analysis than laboratory staff, are often very busy and this is only one of a number of technical processes that they are expected to undertake under pressure. While researchers in Denmark argue that use of PCR testing reduces the number of women given antibiotics in labour (Khalil *et al* 2017), the RCOG noted that, "*The evidence does not suggest that using polymerase chain reaction technology for near-patient testing is feasible in UK maternity ward settings. The technology for near-patient testing continues to improve and it is possible that this may confer benefits in the future.*" (RCOG 2017: e293).

Making bacteriological screening decisions

Women need to make decisions about whether they want to be screened and/or treated for GBS carriage within the context of what is normally offered in their country or area. I will return to a discussion of the wider issues relating to this decision in chapter four, but the following section looks at the factors that need to be weighed up in situations where women are considering being tested for GBS in pregnancy, either because they are in a country that offers bacteriological screening universally, or because they are in a country that does not offer universal culture-based screening but they are considering whether they might want to pursue private testing. In this situation, a number of factors need to be thought through.

What tests are available locally?

The answer to this question will vary depending on where you live, and there is often considerable variation not just between countries but also in different regions of the same country. In the UK for instance, some hospitals only offer GBS testing by the direct plating method and, as above, this method is likely to be used if a swab is being tested because a woman is thought to have an infection rather than because the intention is to specifically test for GBS. But in some areas, it is the only method offered even when the test is specifically intended to look for GBS.

Some hospitals in the UK and elsewhere offer ECM

testing. In some areas ECM testing is available to all women, but some units will offer ECM testing only under certain circumstances, for instance where particular risk factors exist. Some women (and their midwives and doctors; for clinical staff are also at the mercy of policy and guidance) have found that their local hospital or laboratory will carry out an ECM test if specifically asked, but this may not be done routinely or unless specifically requested. As above, at the time of writing, PCR testing for GBS is not commonly used in the UK, though it is in some other countries. Research studies are being carried out in a number of countries and some women will find that they are offered PCR testing within this context.

These factors vary in and between other countries and regions as well. Women living in remote and rural areas have different options than women who live in large cities. The best way of finding out what is available locally is to ask your midwife or doctor. If they don't know, ask them to put you in touch with somebody who can find out for you. This may be another practitioner, the hospital laboratory itself, or a scientist or doctor who works with the laboratory.

Who does the test?

This also depends on where you are and is something you can talk to your midwife or doctor about. Some of the individual studies in this area show that women prefer to collect the swab themselves, while others found that women preferred that a midwife or doctor did the test. I am not going to detail these studies because there is really no question that either of these options are equally good and any woman who decides to have testing should be able to decide which approach is best for her.

Not many guidelines specifically mention this element. In the UK, the RCOG guidance (Hughes *et al* 2017) concludes that, if a woman does decide to have bacteriological testing for some reason, then as long as she is given appropriate instruction, a woman is just as good at collecting her own swab as a midwife or doctor would be. Many women find this less invasive and embarrassing. Details of how this can be done can be found in chapter one of this book, but this process should be fully explained to the woman by the midwife or doctor at the time of the test.

What is the best timing for testing?

It is important not to underestimate the various trade-offs that have to be taken into account if a woman is deciding whether to undergo universal screening for GBS using either the direct plating or ECM test. Although the result is sometimes available faster, both tests can take 2-3 days to complete. Therefore, if a woman wants to know her GBS status before she goes into labour, then she needs to plan to have the test done at least 2-3 days before she is likely to go into labour. This timeframe is not easy to predict and this is one reason why some people view PCR testing as a potentially great advance. As above, there are trade-offs here too, both in financial cost and accuracy.

Another important issue is illustrated by an email I received from a woman who wrote to me from a country which uses PCR testing in labour. She had been distressed by the speed at which she was tested and told that she was carrying GBS bacteria when she arrived at the hospital in labour. She found this quite disconcerting, because she hadn't previously known about the testing. The sample had been taken without her really understanding what it was about or what she was agreeing to. She was then suddenly told that she needed antibiotics in labour a short time after arriving on the labour ward and without having time to properly research this or consider her options. She found this distressing and she felt pressured to agree to have antibiotics at a time when she wasn't really able to process the pros and cons of her decision.

I will return to the wider social elements of this later in the book, but it is important to know that GBS testing is already an area which many women do not feel they were given enough information about beforehand, and offering universal testing in labour may mean that more women end up feeling this way. It is vitally important to consider the impact of asking women to make this kind of decision when they need to focus on being in labour.

Making a decision about when to test may be just as crucial as making the decision about whether to test. Very few women will know when they are going to give birth with any real certainty, and even those who have 'planned' an induction of labour or a caesarean section on a particular date cannot be sure that they won't go into spontaneous labour before that date. So if a woman wants to be tested for GBS, then we might imagine that it makes sense to do it sooner rather than later, to ensure that the result is back before she goes into labour. We also need to bear in mind that occasionally a woman has to be re-tested because a swab didn't contain sufficient material to get a good result or was lost or contaminated during the testing process. It doesn't happen often, but when it does it means re-swabbing and re-testing, which can take another two or three days.

All of this suggests it makes sense to test as early as possible. But this isn't the easy answer that it might seem, because GBS bacteria are transient, by which we mean that they can come and go. So a woman's GBS status can change from day to day or week to week. This means that performing the test too far ahead of the start of labour increases the chance that the test result will not reflect a woman's actual GBS carrier status when she goes into labour. This can happen in both directions, as we saw earlier in the book. Some of the women who test negative for GBS during pregnancy will be carrying GBS when they are in labour, and they won't be offered antibiotics (unless they are in a country that uses risk-based screening and they have a risk factor). In contrast, some of the women who tested positive for GBS will not carry this bacteria by the time they go into labour, but they will still be offered antibiotics and may be told their options are consequently restricted. It is generally accepted that there is no value in testing before 35 weeks of pregnancy and very few women go into labour before this time. NICE (2008) recommend that the collection of cultures between 35 and 37 weeks of gestation appears to achieve the best sensitivity and specificity for identifying women who carry GBS at the time of delivery, although this is based on the results of just one study, carried out in the US (Yancey et al 1996). The researchers in that study estimated that the sensitivity of the 35-37 week test for picking up GBS carriage status at birth was 96%, which means that 4% of women who tested negative between 35 and 37 weeks picked up GBS bacteria before they went into labour. However, 13% (about 1 in 8) of the women who tested positive for GBS at 35-37 weeks were not found to carry GBS when re-tested in labour, although these women would all still have been (unnecessarily) offered antibiotics.

Studies similar to Yancey et al (1996) have since been carried out in the Netherlands (Valkenburg-van den Berg et al 2006), Thailand (Kovavisarach et al 2008) and Portugal (Florindo et al 2014), although the tests women may be offered may differ in some way to the testing methods used in all four of these studies. We also don't know whether changes occur in a woman's vagina when she goes into labour that could affect the test results, but I will return to this question below.

Kovavisarach et al's (2008) findings agreed with those of Yancey et al (1996) in that the 35-37 week test results identified 95.4% of women who tested positive for GBS in labour, but the positive predictive value in this study was even poorer. The testing at 35-37 weeks falsely identified an even greater number of women as carrying GBS in labour with only 70.73% of those identified as carrying GBS at 35-37 weeks having a positive GBS test in labour. This means that just under 30% of the women who were identified as carrying GBS at 35-37 weeks were not considered to be carrying it in labour and would have been offered unnecessary antibiotics and/or found that their birth plans might be affected by this.

In Valkenburg-van den Berg *et al*'s (2006) study, the 35-37 week test wasn't quite as good at identifying women who would carry GBS in labour: it correctly identified 93% of the women who carry GBS in labour. Therefore 7% of women who had a positive GBS test in labour wouldn't have been offered antibiotics. The positive predictive value was 79%, so in this study 21% of women were deemed to be at risk when they had the test but were not identified as carrying GBS by the time they went into labour.

A more recent study in Portugal by Florindo *et al* (2014: 641) compared the results of GBS cultures taken at 35-37 weeks of pregnancy to the results of GBS cultures in labour and found that, *"...of 221 prenatally GBS-positive women, only 54 remained positive at delivery, corresponding to a PPV [or positive predictive value] of 24.4%"*. In other words, 75.6% of women who were found to be carrying GBS at 35-37 weeks of pregnancy were not found to be carrying GBS by the time they gave birth.

This last figure is astonishingly high compared to the results of the other studies previously mentioned. The discrepancy may be partially explained by the fact that women in Portugal choose their own laboratory for screening, which meant that the researchers could not confirm the quality of the sampling, swab storage and testing methods that were used in the 35-37 week screening test. Florindo *et al* (2014) discuss some of the implications of standardisation of GBS detection protocols and screening guidelines, and this may well explain the unusually low positive predictive value.

Even if the magnitude of the difference in Florindo *et al*'s (2014) study is unique to their setting, the general trend is not. *"Both negative (NPV) and positive (PPV) predictive values of prenatal GBS cultures relative to the GBS status at delivery are suboptimal, especially the PPV"* (Florindo *et al* 2014: 640). The difference between the antenatal and in-labour rates of GBS carriage in this research also raises an important point for women who are considering getting their own GBS test done about researching the quality of the testing method.

Women who are thinking about the option of private GBS testing may wish to look into what quality control measures are in place in the laboratories that they are considering, whether and how they are regulated and whether they are offering full and accurate information. It is no secret that an increasing number of commercial companies are offering tests, technologies, drugs and products to pregnant and birthing women and new mothers. Their goal is to make money and websites and adverts may use emotive images, language and stories about highly unusual occurrences in order to generate fear and secure custom. It is always worth doing some research before you make decisions (Wickham 2018a).

The net result of this in all of the studies mentioned here is that, where GBS testing at 35-37 weeks is used as the basis for offering antibiotics in labour, significantly more women will be offered antibiotics. These findings need to be considered in relation to a number of other factors discussed elsewhere in this book and it is probably inevitable that they are interpreted differently, depending on a person's viewpoint. Those who are keen to ensure that they do everything possible to prevent EOGBS disease and are happy to accept the potential costs for both mother and baby (which may be physical, emotional and social as well as financial) of administering more antibiotics than necessary tend to be reassured by the relatively high negative predictive value of testing at 35-37 weeks and see this as the best course of action. Those women who want to be tested and perhaps treated but would rather avoid antibiotics and/or potential restrictions to their birth plans unless they can be more certain that their GBS status is accurate may wish to delay testing. Although we know from these studies that somewhere between 13% and 29.27% (or up to 75.6% if we take Florindo *et al*'s (2014) figures) of the women identified as carrying GBS at 35-37 weeks did not test positive for GBS in labour, we don't have any evidence about whether testing at 38 or 39 weeks would be more accurate. This point was also raised by NICE (2008). We do know, of course, that more women will have gone into labour before that time, so for them the opportunity for testing will have been missed.

The UK RCOG guideline (Hughes *et al* 2017: e209) also suggests that *"If bacteriological tests for GBS are to be performed in pregnancy they should ideally be performed at 35–37 weeks of gestation in order to determine carriage status close to delivery. There is no evidence to support the practice of varying the timing of screening. However, in women where preterm delivery is anticipated, earlier testing is justified."*

Again, this is where accelerated testing is seen as potentially useful. However, it would need to develop to the point where the downsides are reduced and where appropriate, woman-centred information was given before consent is requested.

But there are many things that we don't know. No-one (to the best of my knowledge) has researched whether there is a physiological change in GBS status before and/or during labour. It is possible that there may be a mechanism that prepares a woman's body for labour by 'clearing the way' of bacteria that may be harmful to her baby. Or there may not; we don't know, perhaps because we live in a culture that doesn't prioritise research which considers and celebrates the wisdom of a woman's birthing body. We are really only beginning to understand the human microbiome and the importance of bacteria. If the woman's vagina undergoes changes in order to become more hospitable for her baby to be born, then it is entirely possible that this might include changes in the vaginal flora. The existence of a mechanism to reduce harmful bacteria wouldn't necessarily conflict with the fact that some babies develop EOGBS disease.

A mechanism to provide protection against potentially harmful bacteria may not work as well in some women, for reasons that may be related to genetics, epigenetics, the stage of pregnancy, the environment, their nutritional and/or immunological status or a combination of these or other factors. Would it make a difference if women gave birth at home, in a birth centre or in hospital? What about if they knew all their caregivers? We have no idea. This is all completely speculative as research has not been carried out on these questions. I mention this because I want to keep pointing out that there are many facets of this topic which have thus far been ignored and which may deserve greater attention. I will have more to say about this later in the book.

Private testing

Some women who live in countries that offer risk-based screening decide to undertake private GBS testing. A number of laboratories in the UK and New Zealand offer private ECM testing either by appointment or by post. When the test is done by post, the laboratory sends out the test kit, the woman does the swab test herself and returns the swabs to the laboratory in special packaging. The cost of this testing service in the UK at the time of writing is around £40-£50. The cost of by appointment testing was more variable according to the location and context, but is somewhat higher, as it involves having staff members carrying out the swab test. The organisation *Group B Strep Support* keeps an up-to-date list of laboratories which offer private testing in the UK on its web site at http://gbss.org.uk/what-is-gbs/testing-for-gbs/ecm-test-where-how/

Please also see the resources section in this book to find out how to access information on other organisations that may be able to help you.

Risk-based screening for GBS

The RCOG (Hughes *et al* 2017) and the New Zealand consensus guidelines team (Darlow *et al* 2015) are clearly aware that GBS screening and prophylaxis are controversial. As I have already noted, both provide justification for adopting a risk-based approach to GBS screening and prophylaxis. One of the reasons that the UK has not adopted universal screening is because of studies like that conducted by Oddie and Embleton (2002). These researchers looked at babies who had developed EOGBS disease, and found that 78% of those babies were identifiable through risk factors, such as being born preterm, being born after the waters had been released for more than 18 hours or being born to a woman who had a raised temperature in labour.

This does not mean that all babies who will develop EOGBS disease are identifiable through risk factors alone. Like universal screening, risk-based screening has its limitations. But the idea is that fewer women will be offered antibiotics if the focus is placed on the babies who are potentially at greater risk if they come into contact with GBS bacteria during birth. Let's look in more depth at the categories of babies who are deemed to be at higher risk.

In this section of the book, I'm going to continue to focus on the UK (Hughes *et al* 2017) and New Zealand (Darlow 2015) guidelines, as these are used as the basis for much of the discussion in this area. Guidelines are continually being updated and vary by country and sometimes region, so you may want to check online for the most recent and geographically relevant guidelines to you. This is not hard to do – putting 'group B strep guidelines' and your country or region into a search engine should get you what you need. Or ask your midwife or doctor to point you to a copy of the local guidelines on this topic.

When GBS bacteria are found in risk-based areas

Both the RCOG (Hughes *et al* 2017) and New Zealand (Darlow *et al* 2015) guidance also recommend against universal bacteriological screening. If a woman is found to be carrying GBS (for instance from a urine or vaginal/perianal swab test carried out for another reason, such as investigation of a vaginal discharge), both guidelines recommend that action is taken; this action however, differs.

In the UK, the RCOG recommends that, "*...clinicians should offer IAP to women with GBS bacteriuria identified during the current pregnancy*" (Hughes *et al* 2017: e291). This means that antibiotics will be offered when the woman is in labour. Antibiotic prophylaxis is not offered in pregnancy to women who are found to have GBS on vaginal or anal swabs taken during pregnancy, but oral antibiotics may be offered as treatment to women who are found to have a GBS urinary tract infection during pregnancy. Those women will be offered intravenous antibiotic prophylaxis in labour as well.

The rather obvious implication of this is that, as we have seen, many of the women who are found to carry GBS in pregnancy will not still be carrying the bacteria when they go into labour. This has been addressed in the New Zealand guidance with the recommendation that, "*...women who have had an incidental finding of GBS on a vaginal swab earlier in pregnancy need to [sic] have this repeated between 35–37 weeks. If this has not occurred, then this should be considered a risk factor and she should be offered IAP*" (Darlow *et al* 2015: 70).

A later statement is even stronger: "*An incidental finding of GBS in pregnancy greater than 5 weeks before labour is unreliable and may result in unnecessary intervention in labour*" (Darlow *et al* 2015: 71).

It is not clear why this additional layer has not been added in the UK guidance. I am aware of a number of women in the UK who have requested later testing (after an earlier coincidental finding of GBS, sometimes found without their knowledge that they were being tested) in order to challenge restrictions that have been placed upon them. Most notably the question of whether they would be able to labour and give birth in a midwifery-led unit. The response to their request has been variable.

In some ways, the stance that the RCOG (Hughes *et al* 2017) takes is understandable, especially in the context of our modern culture where doctors and midwives often fear that they may get into legal or professional trouble if they do not 'do as much as possible.' But this element of the guidance can be seen as problematic from both sides of the GBS screening and prophylaxis debate. Those who advocate offering routine laboratory testing for GBS might ask why, if a guideline recommends offering prophylaxis when GBS is found coincidentally, does it not recommend testing everybody? Then there are those who are concerned about the downsides of offering prophylaxis for GBS carriage (whether in general, or just in the absence of other risk factors) and who are pleased that the RCOG has avoided recommending routine screening. Some of these people are confused as to why the RCOG recommends offering antibiotics for GBS carriage found incidentally, especially when it declares elsewhere that the downsides of a policy of universal screening outweigh the benefits. The answer may be that, in maternity care, tradition, fear and/or peer pressure sometimes trump science.

Finally, we need to consider whether women can request GBS testing. In the UK, the RCOG (Hughes *et al* 2017) has recently clarified their position and stated that maternal request alone is not an indication for bacteriological testing on the NHS. However, the fact that the guidelines state that women who are known to be carrying GBS should be offered antibiotics means that women who use a reputable private testing company should not find it difficult to get antibiotics in labour if they are found to be carrying GBS. If women have concerns that they may have a vaginal or urinary tract infection, they will usually find that their midwife or doctor will recommend sending off a swab and/or a mid-stream sample of urine. The tests that are carried out on this may detect the presence of GBS. Again, if they are found to be carrying GBS, the recommendation is that they should be offered antibiotics in labour.

Who is considered at risk in risk-based screening?

Currently, a few groups of babies are deemed to be at risk of being at higher risk of EOGBS disease under risk-based screening guidelines. There is general consensus between the UK and New Zealand guidelines in these areas:

Babies born to women who have been coincidentally found to have GBS bacteria; a situation which we have discussed at length above.

Babies born to women whose waters have released ('broken'). This is a somewhat controversial area and there is some disagreement amongst practitioners here. When a woman who is known to be carrying GBS experiences her waters releasing in the UK, she will be offered antibiotics *"...as soon as reasonably possible"* (Hughes *et al* 2017: e292). This is because we know that the chance of EOGBS disease will increase the longer a woman's waters have been released (Seaward *et al* 1998). However, some UK midwives and doctors believe that, as in New Zealand (Darlow *et al* 2015) and some other countries, it would be better to wait until a woman's waters have been released for 18 hours before offering antibiotics. That is because most women will birth within this timeframe and will not have a baby with EOGBS disease.

Because of the concern about prolonged rupture of membranes being associated with a higher chance of a baby developing GBS disease or another infection, women whose waters release and whose carrier status is unknown will be *"...offered induction immediately or up to 24 hours after*

spontaneous rupture of membranes with unknown carrier status."
(Hughes *et al* 2017: e292).

Of course, women can decide to wait longer. The wider issues surrounding decision making in relation to induction of labour are discussed in more depth in my book *Inducing Labour: making informed decisions* (Wickham 2018b).

Babies born to women who have had a previous baby with EOGBS disease. This is because mothers who have had a previously affected baby are known to have a higher chance of having another affected baby compared to mothers whose babies have not experienced EOGBS disease. *"The reasons for this are not clear but may indicate persistence of carriage or a virulent strain of GBS or a deficient immune response"* (Hughes *et al* 2017: e290).

The main reason for the concern in this area is illustrated by a report of the case of a woman who had two babies with EOGBS disease. The summary of this paper reads:

"At each of two consecutive deliveries a woman gave birth to a baby that developed early-onset group B streptococcal (GBS) septicaemia. A low titre of serum antibodies to the type of the infecting GBS and persistence of the organism in the mother were demonstrated. This case confirms that mothers of GBS infected infants are at high risk of their future babies being similarly infected." (Carstensen *et al* 1988: 201).

Although both babies survived EOGBS disease and went on to be healthy, this paper provided one of the first published discussions of the idea that some babies may be particularly susceptible to EOGBS disease because their mother has a low level of GBS antibodies; as was the case with the woman whose story featured in this paper. Carstensen *et al* (1988: 203) state that, *"...mothers of infants with GBS septicaemia usually have antibody concentrations within or below the lower quarter of the reference area."*

We don't know for sure whether this really is a high-risk situation or whether the woman in question had simply been the unlucky person for whom 'lightning struck twice', but a number of researchers are looking at the question of whether there are even more specific factors which cause some babies to be at higher risk. Studies such as that by Schrag *et al* (2013) which looked at the babies who have EOGBS disease also identify the fact that women had a previous baby with EOGBS disease as a risk factor. But no-one has yet looked more closely at this question of GBS antibodies or managed to quantify the level of this risk (RCOG 2012).

It is hard to understand why researchers haven't sought to better understand this situation, especially as it might be a big clue as to why EOGBS disease only affects a few babies. This seems to be a missed opportunity to find a way of identifying specific women whose babies may be at greater risk. Instead, work is underway to try and develop a vaccine to GBS, although it is unclear how many women would want to have this given the fact that the overall risk of EOGBS disease is low.

It is likely (though not of course inevitable) that women who have previously had a baby with EOGBS disease may already have a strong view on this, which is unlikely to be swayed by evidence. Some women in this situation are very pro antibiotics and pro campaigning. Others have had poor experiences with professionals or consumer campaigning groups during their prior experience and would prefer to avoid intervention as much as possible in future pregnancies. This is a very personal decision.

Babies who are born prematurely. It is not always possible to predict which babies will be born prematurely, so guidance recommends that antibiotics are offered to any woman who appears to be in premature labour (Darlow *et al* 2015, Hughes *et al* 2017). In practice, it can be hard to decide when to offer antibiotics in order to strike a balance between not giving them unnecessarily but starting them early enough so that they will offer some protection to the baby. In many areas, antibiotics are usually offered based on the results of a fetal fibronectin (FFN) test. Although no test is one hundred per cent accurate, this test is a fairly reliable indicator of whether labour will continue.

It is worth noting that this is a recent change in the UK guidance. The previous guidelines (which were published in 2012) stated that antibiotics were not necessary for women in preterm labour whose waters had not released. This guideline stated: *"There is currently no evidence to show that the subgroup of women in preterm labour with ruptured membranes have greater benefit from IAP. The difficulty in balancing risks and benefits of IAP for women in preterm labour could be resolved by a randomised controlled trial."* (RCOG 2012: 4)

Furthermore, there was concern because of the results of a study known as the ORACLE trial (Kenyon *et al* 2001a, Kenyon *et al* 2001b), which was a study set up to look at the effects of giving antibiotics to women who were in preterm labour. The results showed that the babies who had antibiotics were found to have a greater likelihood of adverse neurodevelopmental outcome, including cerebral palsy, and functional impairment at seven years of age, compared to the babies who didn't have antibiotics. The antibiotic used in this trial which caused particular concern (co-amoxiclav) is now no longer used as a result of the ORACLE finding.

The RCOG expressed concern about possible adverse effects of antibiotics where women are in premature labour in its 2012 guideline, recommending that antibiotics were not given unless there were clinical signs of infection. It stated that *"...there is no evidence from long-term follow-up studies that other antibiotics, including penicillin, are safe"* (RCOG 2012: 4). This sentence does not appear in the 2017 guideline (Hughes *et al* 2017). To my knowledge, the reason for their change in guidance was an increase in the incidence of EOGBS disease and the fact that 22% of babies who experienced this were born prematurely. This is again a situation where women may want to weigh up the pros and cons in relation to their individual situation.

Some people have been concerned about whether carrying GBS can increase the chance of preterm labour. This question was considered by Valkenburg-van den Berg *et al* (2009) who undertook a systematic review. They found no association between maternal GBS carriage during pregnancy and preterm delivery.

Babies whose mothers have a higher than normal temperature during labour. A high temperature can be a sign of infection. If a labouring woman has a high temperature, the chance of EOGBS disease is increased (Oddie & Embleton 2002). Women whose temperature is above 38°C in labour will be offered antibiotics in both New Zealand and the UK (Darlow *et al* 2015, Hughes *et al* 2017).

It may also be worth noting that, while it can be very normal for a woman's waters to be released before labour, a raised temperature is not usually normal or benign (except when it has an obvious environmental cause, e.g. it is a very hot day or the woman has been in water which is hotter than ideal) and most midwives and doctors would be concerned about this. A raised temperature can indicate the presence of infection, and because infection can spread more quickly than usual in pregnant and postnatal women and babies, concern is warranted. A raised temperature can sometimes be caused by other things, such as the use of epidural anaesthesia in labour (Wickham 2002). The decision to take antibiotics or not is clearly still up to the woman and needs to be made within the wider context of the situation and any other relevant factors. A woman who has an elevated temperature in labour may, of course, have an infection caused by something other than GBS bacteria. As I noted earlier, GBS isn't a common cause of infection in adults.

Women who were found to be carrying GBS in a previous pregnancy are not considered to be at risk in the same way as the groups discussed above, but the guidance and evidence relating to their situation also needs to be covered here. Research has shown that a woman who has been found to be carrying GBS in one pregnancy has a 40-50% chance of being found to be carrying GBS again in another pregnancy (Tam *et al* 2012, Page-Ramsey *et al* 2013, Coliccia *et al* 2016, Turrentine *et al* 2016). In the UK, the RCOG has recently changed its approach in this area. Previous guidance stated that screening was not indicated for previous GBS carriage alone (RCOG 2013). However, the current revised guidance suggests that in situations where GBS carriage was detected in a previous pregnancy, practitioners should *"Explain to women that the likelihood of maternal GBS carriage in this pregnancy is 50%. Discuss the options of IAP, or bacteriological testing in late pregnancy and the offer of IAP if still positive."* (Hughes *et al* 2017: e290).

The New Zealand guideline does not even mention this; quite possibly because of its stance that any result more than five weeks before labour is unreliable (Darlow *et al* 2015).

The UK guidance goes on to express the change in terms of avoiding over-prescription of antibiotics: *"Assuming that approximately 50% of women will be recurrent carriers, the risk of EOGBS disease should be approximately 2 to 2.5 times that quoted for the total population. The risk of EOGBS disease in the baby in this circumstance is likely to be around 1 in 700 to 1 in 800. At this risk level, some women would choose IAP and others would not. Bacteriological testing in this circumstance would help to refine the risk. A positive bacteriological test in this circumstance would indicate a risk of 1 in 400, but the risk would be 1 in 5000 if the mother is GBS negative. A significant number of mothers may therefore choose to avoid IAP if they test negative."* (Hughes *et al* 2017: e290).

It is again important to remember that, while such an approach may lead to fewer antibiotics being given on a population basis, individual women who agree to have testing and are found to be carrying GBS may find their decisions are restricted as a result. Where this happens, the fact that the recommendation may lead to an overall reduction in antibiotic prescription may not feel reassuring.

A few notes on risk-based screening

There are a few specific situations which are worth discussing here because, although they may not be considered as risk factors, enough women and clinicians have questions about them that they are mentioned in one or other of the key guidelines in this area.

Treating GBS colonisation in pregnancy. Even if GBS bacteria are found on a vaginal or anal swab during pregnancy, antibiotics are not recommended at the time unless there are signs of infection (Hughes *et al* 2017). This element of GBS guidance is fairly uncontroversial, and there are number of reasons behind this element of the guidelines.

(1) Antibiotics will be offered in labour anyway, so offering them in pregnancy would mean extra doses.

(2) Even if antibiotics were given in pregnancy, the GBS bacteria could return before labour.

(3) The baby is not considered to be in any danger from GBS during pregnancy, as it is protected within the bag of membranes which contains amniotic fluid.

(4) Offering antibiotics in pregnancy would further increase the problem of antibiotic overuse.

A number of recent papers have expressed concern about the percentage of pregnant women who receive antibiotics in pregnancy (Adriaenssens *et al* 2011, Broe *et al* 2014, Braye *et al* 2017). In my research on this area, I haven't encountered anyone who argues against this point.

If a woman has symptoms of a vaginal infection in pregnancy (such as a high temperature and/or pulse, or vaginal discharge) or if GBS is found in a urine sample, this is a different matter; antibiotics are offered to treat those symptoms. If a woman had been found to carry GBS and was treated in pregnancy because she had symptoms of an infection, she would still be offered antibiotics in labour because of the possibility that the GBS could return.

GBS and induction of labour. If a woman decides to have her labour induced, the induction methods that are available to her are not affected by her GBS status (Hughes *et al* 2017). Hughes *et al* (2017) also state that membrane sweeping (also known as 'stretching and sweeping'), which is offered to many women as an early element of the induction process, is not contraindicated in women who have GBS bacteria. This is based on a small study conducted by Kabiri *et al* (2015). Some experts feel that more research is needed in the area of vaginal examination (which is a necessary part of membrane sweeping) and GBS.

GBS and waterbirth. GBS status does not preclude using water for labour and/or birth (Hughes *et al* 2017). However, some women in the UK and elsewhere have found they are told they cannot use a hospital or birth centre pool if they are found to have GBS. Of course, they can stay at home and get a pool of their own, and some do this, but others want to be able to use a pool in the birthing facility of their choice. Any woman who finds herself in this situation in the UK might find it useful to refer caregivers to this element of the RCOG guidance. There is more on this topic in the 'frequently asked questions' section of this book. The organisation Birthrights also has information on women's rights during labour and birth and you can find more information on this and other organisations in the resources section.

GBS and planned caesarean. Women who are planning caesarean and whose membranes are intact will not be offered antibiotics specifically for GBS. But this statement can be confusing, because all women who have a caesarean will be given antibiotics just before or during the operation, unless they specifically request otherwise, as women are generally not consulted separately about antibiotics when consenting for surgery. This is because consent for surgery will assume consent for an entire package of care and associated interventions, including intravenous antibiotics.

This has been rightly questioned (Anonymous author 2017) but it may be some time before practice changes.

However, these routinely given antibiotics are for the benefit of the woman rather than the baby, because caesareans carry a chance of infection. Also, as they are given just before or during the operation this is not deemed soon enough to be beneficial for the baby. There is a question however about whether or not giving intravenous antibiotics before the cord is clamped (and some antibiotics are transferred to the baby) may have unwanted consequences, such as affecting the baby's microbiome.

Although the RCOG (2012, Hughes *et al* 2017) does not discuss the thinking behind this part of the guideline, it may have a practical basis, as it would be difficult to be able to time antibiotics effectively in women having planned caesareans, which are frequently delayed or postponed. In addition, the babies of women having planned caesareans may also be deemed to be at low risk of developing EOGBS disease where they are being born at term and the membranes are intact. Women who are having a planned caesarean and who want to have antibiotics that may also offer protection against EOGBS disease may wish to discuss this with their midwife or doctor.

GBS and unplanned caesarean. Women who have an unplanned caesarean and who have spent at least some time in labour may have already been offered antibiotics for their baby if their baby was deemed to be at risk. The NICE (2011) guidance on antibiotics for caesarean section means that women having an unplanned caesarean will also be offered antibiotics for their own benefit. As this is a complex area, if women know they carry GBS and are very keen to have a particular antibiotic, they may wish to discuss ahead of time what would happen if they needed an unplanned caesarean in labour. This would also apply if a woman had an allergy or a previous reaction to a particular antibiotic.

How were the risk factors determined?

I am sometimes asked how guideline writers in the countries using a risk-based approach came up with the risk factors which would identify which women/babies were offered antibiotics. The answer is that they were based on studies which looked at the babies who developed EOGBS disease, in order to see whether this was at all predictable. The first of these studies was published in the British Medical Journal by Oddie and Embleton in 2002. This is a fairly well-known and often-cited study in the field, because the authors made the case for a risk-based approach to GBS screening in the UK rather than testing every woman for GBS. The authors wanted to find out how common EOGBS disease was, and to see if they could identify any particular risk factors. They collected details of babies who developed EOGBS disease in one area of Northern England and compared these babies with matched babies who did not have EOGBS disease. In total, 36 babies developed EOGBS disease out of a total of 62,786. This is 1 in 1744 babies.

Oddie and Embleton's (2002) findings included the discovery that premature babies (those born before 37 completed weeks of pregnancy) comprised 38% of all cases of EOGBS disease, and 83% (5 out of 6) of the babies who died from EOGBS disease had been born before 36 completed weeks of pregnancy. They found that 68% of the babies with EOGBS disease were born to women whose waters had released more than 18 hours before they were born. And 19% of the babies with EOGBS disease were born to women who had a temperature in labour. This is why midwives and doctors do not assume GBS infection when a woman has a high temperature in labour and also why, if antibiotics are offered to treat suspected maternal infection, they are more likely to be broad-spectrum antibiotics rather than the narrow-spectrum benzyl penicillin which is the antibiotic of choice when we want to specifically target GBS bacteria.

These findings were echoed by those of the NeonIN surveillance network (Vergnano *et al* 2011), which carried out research to look at the pattern of neonatal infection in twelve neonatal units in England over a two-year period from 2006-2008. While Vergnano *et al* (2011) looked at all causes of infection, and not just GBS, they found that GBS was responsible for more infections than any other bacteria. It is important to know that, in practice, we can't always determine which bacteria caused an illness or infection. The finding that GBS caused more infections than any other bacteria is, as I mentioned near the beginning of this book, one reason why GBS receives so much attention, even though the absolute number of babies affected is very small. Vergnano *et al* (2011) also discovered that the majority of neonatal infections occurred in babies who were born before 37 completed weeks of pregnancy and/or who had low birthweight of less than 2500g, with 82% and 81% of babies being in each of these categories, respectively.

Similar studies continue to inform each iteration of the guidelines that are produced, and this is one reason that guidance changes over time. It is worth knowing, however, that surveillance and similar data are hard to collect accurately, although researchers go to a lot of trouble to look into as many cases as possible.

We need to bear two other things in mind here. First, most women who have a risk factor will not have a baby with EOGBS disease. In fact, very few of the women in these situations will have babies who become affected by EOGBS disease, which is why even a risk-based approach leads to significant overtreatment with antibiotics. It is simply that population-level studies have helped identify the babies who are at greater risk and offer an alternative to universal screening.

Secondly, babies born to women who do not carry GBS are not likely to get EOGBS disease, even if they are born prematurely or a long time after the waters have released. If only 20% of women are carrying GBS bacteria at any given time, that means that 80% of women whose babies are deemed to be at higher risk of EOGBS disease under the UK and NZ guidelines will not be at risk of EOGBS disease. Yet their mothers are also being offered antibiotics. This is one reason that some people call for a combination of the two approaches, as I discussed earlier in the book.

All that population-level studies can do is to suggest factors that may indicate that a baby is at higher risk. Women and their families then need to decide what they think and feel about their own situation in the light of this data and other information.

Other possible risk factors

The Cochrane review in this area lists other risk factors that have found to be correlated with an increased chance of a baby developing EOGBS disease. These have generally not been considered in the UK (RCOG 2012, Hughes *et al* 2017) or New Zealand (Darlow *et al* 2015) guidance and it is not hard to imagine why from even a brief analysis of these factors. First, much of the research has been carried out in countries other than the UK, which makes it hard to know whether the issues would necessarily be the same here. Most of the papers cited below are reporting on single studies, and the results may not be significant or reliable enough in themselves. But even more important is the fact that, in some cases, there is nothing that we can really do with the information before the baby is born, other than perhaps cause women unnecessarily anxiety, stress or concern.

For example, research by Baker and Barrett (1973), Dillon *et al* (1987), Schuchat (1999), and Yagupsky *et al* (1991) identified that EOGBS disease was more likely in babies who weighed less than 2500g at birth. While this might be helpful knowledge once a baby is born, we have no completely accurate way of predicting birthweight before birth, so there is little we can do with this information. In any case, many babies who are under this birthweight will also be preterm; a situation which is already covered by the RCOG guidelines. A study by Schuchat (1999) in the USA identified black women, teenagers and women who have previously had a miscarriage to be at higher risk. More recently, Spiel *et al* (2019) found that African American women were more likely to convert to carrying GBS in the last few weeks of pregnancy than non-Hispanic white women: 9.2% as compared to 5.3% (Spiel *et al* 2019). We have no idea why this might be. A South African study suggested that babies born to women with HIV may be more susceptible to EOGBS (le Doare *et al* 2015). Finally, Håkansson and Källén (2006) found that women with gestational diabetes were at higher risk but, again, this was not the finding of similar studies which involved UK women. The different definitions of and treatments for gestational diabetes between countries may account for this difference.

We do not know exactly what percentage of UK women would be offered antibiotics within the current guidelines (that is, if they were followed 'to the letter' in practice). It is also of note that the number of women who are deemed to be at risk depends a lot on how many women are deemed to need a swab or urine test for other reasons in pregnancy. It is also influenced by the proportion of women who undertake private GBS testing, so there will likely always be considerable variation between areas and over time.

The consequences of knowledge

As you may have gathered, although some countries don't recommend routine screening, many guidelines and practitioners are quick to recommend or even encourage antibiotics when a woman has been found to carry GBS. Often, as I have previously discussed, that finding is the coincidental result of a test to investigate possible infection in the woman.

This situation is worth bearing in mind if you are considering whether or not to have screening, especially in view of the previously stated fact that a significant proportion of women who test positive at 35-37 weeks won't be carrying GBS when they go into labour. In New Zealand, you should be offered screening again, but in the UK an early finding of GBS may affect your experience throughout pregnancy, labour and birth. Your care may not change during pregnancy, but you may find you are told that your labour and birth options have changed as a result of a positive test result. I know of several cases where a woman in the UK had a negative GBS test in late pregnancy following an earlier positive test but was still put under immense and unwanted pressure to have antibiotics when she was in labour. Women in some areas describe being 'cajoled' and even 'bullied' into accepting prophylaxis.

There is an important point here. Once you have a GBS screening test, you can't 'unknow' the results of this test, and neither can you remove it from your medical records (Wickham 2009). Women can find that they are under a lot of pressure to have screening and prophylaxis for GBS; not just from professionals, but sometimes from their family, other women, consumer groups and even information helplines. Women may want to think through whether or not they would want antibiotics in labour before deciding whether or not to have testing. I receive a lot of emails from women who feel that some of the GBS support groups are actually only supportive of the idea that all women should have antibiotics in labour.

Many women do not realise that this situation is different from some of the other tests that are offered in pregnancy. With most antenatal screening tests for instance, you will be offered the option of having a test or not and it will be up to you to make the decision. Your decision will usually be respected either way. In the case of GBS screening, the decision is still up to you, but women in countries which offer universal screening are often put under pressure to accept this testing, and some women in countries like the UK that use risk-based screening have found that some of the information is geared towards persuading them to have a GBS test done privately. Some of this information comes from companies who profit from selling private GBS testing. Furthermore, women who have risk factors or who decide to be screened and are found to carry GBS are often put under significant pressure to have antibiotics in labour. Much of the GBS literature given out in clinics and hospitals is biased towards having antibiotics in labour and many women have found it to be 'fear-based' rather than balanced. As mentioned previously, the decision also has implications in relation to where women are able to give birth, in that they might be denied admission to a midwife-led birth centre if it does not have facilities for giving intravenous antibiotics. Some women who have said that they do not wish to have antibiotics in labour have been told that they are still not 'allowed' to birth there, because the unit is not set up to deal with affected babies. This seems odd, because every midwife-led birth centre occasionally experiences an unexpected problem or situation and they have clear guidelines and referral pathways to deal with these. So these are all things to bear in mind as you decide what is right for you.

Finally, as was pointed out in a previous edition of the UK NICE (2008) guideline, no research has been carried out to compare antenatal screening with no screening; that is, to see if more babies are saved when women are screened. Nor have any trials been undertaken to compare different screening strategies. Current guidance continues to recommend that *"Pregnant women should not be offered routine antenatal screening for group B streptococcus because evidence of its clinical and cost effectiveness remains uncertain"* (NICE 2019).

As we will discuss in the next section of the book, there are quite a few studies showing correlations (or relationships) between the introduction of GBS-related screening and prophylaxis strategies and a reduction in the number of babies who develop EOGBS disease. However, there are a number of things we need to consider when looking at this kind of research, and their results may not be as reliable as some people may think.

There are no rights and wrongs here. The important thing is to weigh up the information, consider your own circumstances, beliefs and feelings and to make the best decision that you can for your own personal situation.

3. GBS Prophylaxis

While approaches to determining whose babies are at risk from EOGBS disease differ widely between countries, most maternity care systems have policies clearly stating that, where an unborn baby is thought to be at risk, the most appropriate response is to offer prophylactic (preventative) intravenous antibiotics to its mother during labour.

Intravenous antibiotics are thought to help in this situation in two ways. First, it is hoped that they will eliminate the GBS bacteria from the woman's vagina, so that they cannot be transferred to her baby during birth. Secondly, as intravenous antibiotics cross the placenta, they will be in the baby's system when it is born and it is hoped that they may help treat any GBS infection that the baby has acquired.

All antibiotics come with downsides, risks and side effects, and not everyone wants to take them (or give them to a baby) unless they are really necessary and there is actual evidence of infection. The consequences of screening and being deemed to be at risk also have implications for women and families. As the RCOG guideline notes:

"A positive antenatal screen will result in the recommendation of IAP which carries some risks for the mother and baby. These include anaphylaxis, increased medicalisation of labour and the neonatal period, and possibly, infection with antibiotic-resistant organisms when broad-spectrum antibiotics, such as amoxicillin, are used for prophylaxis." (Hughes *et al* 2017: e286)

Some women who have a risk factor or who have found they carry GBS decide to do nothing except keep a close eye on their baby once she or he is born; especially during the first 24 hours when EOGBS disease is most likely to manifest. Other women decide to have the intravenous antibiotic prophylaxis offered within systems of maternity care, while others use alternative approaches in an attempt to remove or reduce harm from any GBS bacteria.

When women decide to have intravenous antibiotics, the current recommendation from the RCOG (Hughes *et al* 2017) is that:

"For women who have agreed to IAP, benzyl penicillin should be administered. Once commenced, treatment should be given regularly until delivery. It is recommended that 3 g intravenous benzyl penicillin be given as soon as possible after the onset of labour and 1.5 g 4-hourly until delivery.*"* (Hughes *et al* 2017: e292-93)

Many areas of the world recommend a similar type and dosage of antibiotic, although the New Zealand guideline recommends a smaller dose of *"intravenous benzyl penicillin. Initial dose 1.2g and then 0.6g, 4 hourly until birth."* (Darlow *et al* 2015: 73).

A really important recent change in some guidelines relates to the recommendation of which antibiotic should be given to women who wish to have prophylaxis but who are allergic to penicillin. Previously, the UK recommendation was to give an antibiotic called Clindamycin. However, this *"...can no longer be recommended as the current resistance rate in the UK [is] 16%"* (Hughes *et al* 2017: e296). The NZ guidelines also mention antibiotic resistance (Darlow *et al* 2015), and it is a really stark reminder of why we should be really concerned about antibiotic overuse. The risk of giving prophylactic antibiotics to tens of thousands of people who do not need them is that those antibiotics will not be effective in the future for other people who really do need them for the treatment of an infection.

Before I look at the evidence and other issues relating to antibiotics in more depth, I want to explain what having antibiotics in labour entails for a woman who decides to take this path. Apart from anything else, this enables me to define and explain some of the terminology at the outset.

When women have antibiotics in labour

If a woman decides to have antibiotics in labour, these will be given directly into her bloodstream (intravenously, or via a 'drip') through a small plastic tube (also known as a cannula, Venflon or Luer) which is inserted into a vein in her hand or wrist. Although it is possible to get oral antibiotics (which are taken by mouth as tablets), these are not considered to be effective enough in the case of EOGBS disease prevention in labour. We will consider whether intravenous antibiotics are effective below.

The intravenous cannula will be inserted by a midwife or doctor by means of a special introducer needle which is removed as soon as the tube has been inserted. It is usually inserted once the woman is considered to be in established labour. 'Established labour' is a frustrating term used by midwives and doctors to describe when they think that the woman's labour has reached the point where they feel it is going to carry on until the baby is born. This can sometimes feel confusing and annoying for a woman because it doesn't account for the hours of labour that she may have experienced before this point, and it is one of those definitions which have little or no meaning within the more important context of the woman's experience.

One situation in which the starting point to give antibiotics is a bit more defined is where a woman is having her labour induced. In this situation, the first dose of antibiotics will usually be given at the onset of the Syntocinon (or Pitocin) drip which is used to stimulate contractions (see Wickham 2018b). This is particularly the case where women have already had one or more babies. The antibiotics are started at this point to increase the chance that antibiotics will have been given for at least four hours before the birth.

A skilled midwife or doctor can usually insert a cannula quickly, although it can be painful, especially as it may be difficult for a woman to stay still through the sensations of labour. In many countries, the standard of care is that, if a woman has a cannula inserted before or during labour, a fairly large gauge cannula is used. This is because, if the woman has excessive bleeding after the birth, a larger cannula means that fluids or blood can be replaced more quickly. If a woman decides to have antibiotics but does not like needles, she may wish to let her midwife know this. The woman can ask for a smaller cannula or for the procedure to be performed by someone who is experienced.

In most areas, a blood sample is taken when a cannula is inserted, most often as a precautionary measure in case the woman needs a blood transfusion later. Women can ask what this blood will be tested for and let the midwife or doctor know if they do not wish for this to happen. As with any intravenous procedure, there is a risk of infection from the cannula site, although this is rare. Other risks of having intravenous antibiotics are discussed below.

The antibiotics are prescribed by a midwife or doctor and will usually be given by the person caring for the woman in labour. There are two main ways of giving the antibiotics: the first dose is usually put in a small bag of saline fluid which is hung up on a drip pole or machine while it drips down into the woman's arm through the cannula. This usually takes 15 to 20 minutes. The second and subsequent doses may be given in the same way, or they may be put in a syringe and given by slow injection directly into the cannula in the woman's arm. This is sometimes referred to as a bolus. With this method, it usually takes about five minutes for the drugs to be slowly injected into the cannula, and then the syringe can be removed.

Because most guidelines recommend that antibiotics continue to be given throughout labour, at four or six-hourly intervals until the baby is born, the cannula will often be left in for the rest of the woman's labour. It should not be continually attached to a drip though, unless intravenous fluids are being given for other reasons, for instance because the woman's labour has been induced or augmented (artificially speeded up) with a drug such as Syntocinon. When the cannula is inserted, it should be carefully covered with a special dressing (plaster) so that the woman can move freely without fearing that she will bang or catch the cannula on something and hurt her hand or dislodge the cannula.

Women who do not need a cannula for other reasons can ask for a small gauge cannula to be used and for this to be removed between doses of antibiotics if they prefer. One situation where this approach is deemed preferable by many midwives is where the woman wants to have a shower, bath or use a birth pool. Removing the cannula in between doses reduces the chance of an infection, especially in the pool, as well as being more comfortable, but a few women prefer to ask for the cannula to be covered and kept in rather than having another one sited later in their labour. There are also situations when a woman may decide to keep the cannula in based on the recommendation of a caregiver, but having a cannula in place does not mean that a woman should be denied access to a pool for labour or birth. The cannula can be covered with a glove or plastic bag and a bandage may be helpful to keep this in place and allow the woman to relax and not worry about whether it will get wet.

If it has only been used for antibiotics (and not other fluids or drugs) and the woman has not had any problems (such as excessive bleeding) the cannula will usually be removed as soon as the woman has given birth. Some women are asked to wait until they have been to the toilet and/or are ready to shower, but a woman can ask for it to be removed at any time. The cannula needs to be removed carefully, as it is in vein which may bleed, and it will need to have pressure put on it for a short while after it is removed. Occasionally, a woman may develop a bruise after having a cannula, and the site may feel tender.

Local variation in antibiotic prophylaxis

Every country that has a guideline relating to GBS tends to recommend a particular antibiotic of choice when women decide to have prophylaxis, with alternatives where women who decide to have antibiotics have an allergy to the kind that is usually offered. Many hospitals have their own guideline as well.

In reality, the antibiotic recommended in the national or local guideline is not always the antibiotic that is given. This is an area in which local protocols frequently differ from national guidance and midwives and doctors who attend my courses frequently report that the policy or practice in their unit or area differs from what is recommended in their country. There are sometimes even differences between practitioners working in the same hospital. This has also been confirmed by research (Briody *et al* 2016).

In most countries, the recommended antibiotic for GBS prophylaxis is penicillin. Penicillin is a narrow-spectrum antibiotic known to be effective against GBS. 'Narrow-spectrum' means that an antibiotic is effective only against a limited range of bacteria and this contrasts from broad-spectrum antibiotics which are effective against a broader range of organisms.

Most frequently, 3g of penicillin is initially given as an infusion, with subsequent doses of 1.5g via bolus. The antibiotic given to women who decide to have antibiotics but have a penicillin allergy varies between different areas. Women who decide they want to have antibiotics may wish to ask which antibiotic would be given ahead of time.

If you are hoping that I am going to tell you which antibiotic is most effective, then I am sadly going to disappoint you. As the RCOG (2012) note, *'dosage regimens are based on tradition rather than evidence'*, which may also explain some of these differences. Edwards *et al* (2015) discovered significant variation in the beliefs and practices of US-based obstetricians in this area. Despite these deviations, most local guidelines are clear that broad spectrum antibiotics such as ampicillin should be avoided where possible. There are other reasons to not recommend certain types of antibiotics. For example, clinicians in the UK are advised not to use clindamycin because of high rates of antibiotic resistance (Hughes *et al* 2017). The overuse of antibiotics, especially broad spectrum antibiotics, is causing some kinds of bacteria to become resistant to the antibiotics, and there is a need to save these for situations when they are needed to treat people who have an actual infection rather than overusing them as a preventative measure.

Antibiotics: the dimensions of effectiveness

Probably the most important question that we need to consider in this section of the book is: do antibiotics work? Are they effective at preventing EOGBS disease in babies?

Unfortunately, the answer to that isn't as straightforward as we might like, as I will explain over the next few pages. If I had to summarise what we currently know at this point in time in three words, they would be: *We don't know.*

The reason we don't know is that we don't have good enough research data. The reason that we don't have good enough research data is that we haven't run large enough trials of appropriate quality to be able to effectively measure the effectiveness of antibiotics to prevent EOGBS disease. The reason we haven't run those trials is, as I said in chapter two, many maternity care recommendations and practices are based on tradition or belief and not science.

This situation is summarised by the authors of the largest and best-respected medical review in this area:

"Ideally the effectiveness of IAP to reduce neonatal GBS infections should be studied in adequately sized double-blind controlled trials.

The opportunity to conduct such trials has likely been lost, as practice guidelines (albeit without good evidence) have been introduced in many jurisdictions." (Ohlsson & Shah 2014: 1)

So although we don't have good evidence from clinical trials that antibiotics work, these are still offered to women whose babies are perceived to be at risk of EOGBS disease because this has become the standard of care despite the lack of reliable or robust research evidence. A full explanation of why this is the case is beyond the scope of this book, but much of the reason for this relates to the way our culture views health, responsibility and what people can expect from midwives, doctors and systems of health care. Some practitioners feel that they would rather do something (even if it's not necessarily effective and even if it has side effects) than nothing, and some parents feel the same way. Others are scared that they might be blamed or even sued if they don't do everything possible. It is *doing* that is the key word here. So often, in health care and other areas, it is deemed better to *do* something 'just in case' than to wait and watch what happens, acting only if there is a genuine problem. Many people have questioned the wisdom of this approach.

Interventions can sometimes spread because people are wary of not doing what the doctor or hospital up the road is doing, even if what they are doing isn't based on good evidence. Over time, once a few people or places are doing something (like recommending antibiotics because a baby is deemed to be at risk from GBS) it soon becomes a norm and an expectation. It is then difficult for professionals not to recommend it, as they have historically been judged against what other professionals do, sometimes instead of what the evidence says. Standard practice can be difficult to oppose.

That said, there are a few studies of lesser quality that indicate that antibiotics may be effective at reducing GBS carriage, but I will return to a discussion of those in a moment. First, I want to explain more about the review above, which entails a brief discussion about how we measure the effectiveness of medical interventions.

Measuring effectiveness in research

There are lots of different ways in which research can be undertaken and all have their place, but if you want to measure the effectiveness of a drug at treating a particular disease, then it is very well accepted within science and medicine that the best way to do this is by carrying out a randomised controlled trial (RCT), ideally a double-blind RCT which is considered to be the 'gold standard'. In this kind of study, you take a group of people, randomly divide them into two (or sometimes more) groups, and give one group the intervention and the other group a placebo that 'looks, smells, tastes and feels' like the intervention. Then you watch and measure what happens in each group. The reason for having a placebo is because when someone gives us a pill, sometimes we get better because we think we'll get better. This is called the placebo effect and, in a well-designed trial, neither the woman nor her caregiver knows who has had the real drug and who has had the placebo. When a placebo is used in this way, it is called a double blind trial (because neither the woman nor her midwife or doctor knows who is having the real drug. Single blind means that the caregiver knows but the woman doesn't.)

In these kind of trials, we need to be very clear and specific about what we think a drug will do and have a very measurable outcome. For instance, and I apologise for the starkness of this example but it is the reality of medical research, we might decide we are going to count the number of babies who die or who suffer from a particular problem after getting a disease. In this scenario, the researchers need to be very clear about how the disease is defined and diagnosed. We have already seen that testing isn't one hundred per cent accurate, and the symptom pictures of different diseases can often look very similar, so all of these things need to be considered very carefully. Also, because diseases such as EOGBS disease are thankfully rare, a research study that was going to include mortality (death) as an outcome would need to randomise a lot of women and babies to see whether there was a statistically significant difference between antibiotic prophylaxis and the placebo.

One important reason that we need well-designed research studies is because the changes in the incidence and outcomes of problems like EOGBS disease can be caused by a number of factors, which means we cannot just rely on counting what happens at different times and assuming that a particular programme or intervention that was introduced is the cause of the difference. Many factors can affect the health of women and babies, including nutrition, a woman's smoking status and whether she or her baby are over or under average weight. Then there are demographic or social factors, such as poverty, ethnicity or migration status.

Any change which occurs over a particular time period may be due to changes in maternity care, to the screening and/or prophylaxis which is being offered specifically in relation to GBS, to the number of antibiotics that women are taking for reasons unrelated to GBS or perhaps other factors that I have not listed here. Although some people will argue that change in the rates of EOGBS disease over time is due to the screening and prophylaxis offered, this is not a given, and I have listed some of the other possible factors here in order to illustrate just how much about this area (and, indeed, many other areas of maternity care) is still unknown.

These are just some of the reasons that we need to have good ways of measuring the effectiveness of different kinds of screening and prophylaxis. Hopefully, my explanation of the complexities of a research trial will go part of the way to explain why it is not always straightforward to find the answer to questions such as whether antibiotics are effective at reducing the mortality rate from EOGBS disease. But let's look at the review of the trials that have been carried out in this area, as that will explain it further.

The Cochrane review

The Cochrane Collaboration has published several versions of a review of the trials which have been carried out *"...to assess the effect of intrapartum antibiotics for maternal Group B haemolytic streptococci (GBS) colonization on mortality from any cause, from GBS infection and from organisms other than GBS"* (Ohlsson & Shah 2014: 1). The authors describe the importance of reviewing the trials in this area thus:

"It is important to know if intrapartum antibiotics do more good than harm in trying to reduce mortality and morbidity from neonatal GBS infections. Most women colonized with GBS are asymptomatic [without symptoms of infection], so screening is necessary if these women are to be identified. However, of the women in labor who are GBS positive, very few will give birth to babies who are infected with GBS. Hence, giving IV antibiotics to all women in labor who are GBS positive will put a large number of women and babies at risk of adverse effects unnecessarily. These adverse effects include potentially fatal anaphylaxis, increase in drug-resistant organisms and the medicalization of labor and the neonatal period." (Ohlsson & Shah 2014: 4).

Ohlsson and Shah (2014) set out to see if antibiotics worked for <u>known</u> [my emphasis] *group B strep colonisation*. I am underlining this because I want to highlight the slipperiness of the word *known* in this situation. First, only women who live in countries like the US or Australia which offer routine screening and women who actively choose to have GBS screening will *know* if they were carrying GBS when they were tested or not. But we have to bear in mind that the tests aren't totally accurate, and that GBS carriage status may change. Some women who *know* (or think they know) they carry GBS actually won't have it, and some women will think they *know* that they don't have it when they actually do.

Another concern is that the review didn't set out to look at the effectiveness of antibiotics in countries like the UK and New Zealand which offer antibiotics when women have risk factors or who have be found to be carrying GBS on a screening test. These countries, as we have seen, do not offer universal GBS testing to all women. Women in countries using risk-based screening aren't really at a disadvantage here though, because the reviewers didn't find much good evidence for universal screening anyway. Despite searching on a global scale, Ohlsson and Shah (2014) identified only four relevant randomised controlled trials which met their criteria for the review. Many more trials have been carried out, but they were rejected for one or more reasons, mostly because that they weren't of good enough quality to generate results that could be trusted.

The trials that were included in the 2014 review were published between 1986 and 2002. Three of the included trials involved a total of 500 women and evaluated the effect of antibiotics versus no antibiotics. However, none of these studies used blinding, and for this and several other reasons they were considered to be at high risk for potential bias. That is, their findings cannot be considered reliable. The fourth trial, involving a total of 352 women, compared two different antibiotics: penicillin and ampicillin. It is not clear whether women and their caregivers were blinded to which antibiotic they had. This trial was considered to be of somewhat better quality than the other three, but as it did not include a control group of women who did not have an antibiotic, its results do not help answer the question of whether antibiotics are more effective than a placebo.

Ohlsson and Shah (2014) went on to analyse and present the results of the trials, although they repeatedly point out that they do not consider the data to be trustworthy because the trials were flawed in several respects:

"The use of IAP did not significantly reduce the incidence of all cause mortality, mortality from GBS infection or from infections caused by bacteria other than GBS. The incidence of early GBS infection was reduced with IAP compared to no treatment (risk ratio (RR) 0.17, 95% confidence interval (CI) 0.04 to 0.74, three trials, 488 infants; risk difference -0.04, 95% CI -0.07 to -0.01;

80

number needed to treat to benefit 25, 95% CI 14 to 100, I² 0%)." (Ohlsson & Shah 2014: 1-2).

In lay terms this means that antibiotics seem to decrease the number of babies who developed GBS infection but the antibiotics made no difference to the numbers of babies who died, whether from EOGBS disease or another infection. The small number of women included in the trials makes it rather unlikely that these data would show a difference in mortality anyway. This is one of the things that Ohlsson and Shah (2014) have to say about the untrustworthiness of these findings:

"It is remarkable that in North America the commonly implemented practice of IAP to GBS colonized women has been so poorly studied. Only three randomized controlled trials conducted more than 20 years ago in three different countries and enrolling a total of 500 women have been published. We identified serious concerns of bias in these trials affecting our ability to draw conclusions from this systematic review. Concerns include no preset sample sizes, the lack of a placebo in the control groups, women and care-providers not blinded to group assignment, reporting on outcomes while the trials were ongoing, and exclusion of women who developed signs of infections in labor." (Ohlsson & Shah 2014: 14)

Understandably, this situation leaves many parents and practitioners feeling confused and frustrated. There is no good randomised controlled trial data to show us whether antibiotics have any effect on reducing the number of babies who die or become sick from EOGBS disease. There is a desperate need for good randomised controlled trials in this area, because we genuinely don't know whether antibiotics work to reduce mortality (death) and/or morbidity (illness) from EOGBS disease or not. However, the entrenched nature of obstetric practices such as this within a risk-focused culture mean that many people believe it would be impossible to run the research trials that would generate this knowledge. The alternative to running trials is to continue to use risk screening and offer prophylaxis which we hope might work but whose effectiveness is unknown and which we do know can be harmful.

Other research on antibiotics and GBS carriage

A significant number of other studies have been carried out and published in this area. I will look at some of their results here, but it is important to reiterate that most of these are not randomised controlled trials, and thus are not the best kind of research to use to evaluate the effectiveness of antibiotic prophylaxis. I am not going to look further at the randomised controlled trials that Ohlsson and Shah (2014) rejected from their analysis, because they are of even less use in answering our questions than those already discussed.

The reason that these other kinds of studies are not ideal is because there are so many places where bias can enter the frame, which can mean that the results and any conclusions we draw from the results might be wrong. Any kind of knowledge, including that derived from research findings, needs to be considered in context. In this section I will offer a bit more contextual information about what we can and cannot learn from different kinds of studies.

Ohlsson and Shah (2014: 4) offer a good overview of the state of the rest of the science:

"Although these current guidelines are based on studies of poor quality (Ohlsson & Mhyr 1994), there seems to be a temporal association between the introduction of guidelines and a decline in the GBS EOD [early onset disease] rate (CDC 2005; CDC 2007; Schrag et al 2002). The incidence of invasive early-onset GBS disease decreased from 1.8 cases/1000 live births in the early 1990s to 0.26 cases/1000 live births in 2010 (Schrag et al 2013). However, there has been no reduction in LOD [or late onset] GBS disease in infants (CDC 2007; Schrag et al 2013). Mortality has decreased. The same literature has been interpreted differently by different professional organizations. All cases of EOD cannot be prevented."

The fact that the literature has been interpreted differently in different areas is very telling, as it reflects the fact that the research findings are not clear-cut. The study by Schrag *et al* (2002), for instance, is often quoted by groups promoting screening for GBS carriage and antibiotic prophylaxis in the hope of reducing the chance of a baby developing EOGBS disease. This was a large retrospective cohort study, and these researchers concluded that screening (and, as a consequence, antibiotic prophylaxis) reduced the rate of EOGBS disease. However, they measured the effectiveness of this to be in the region of 86-89%, so a proportion of babies still developed EOGBS disease despite their mothers having had the recommended screening and/or antibiotics in labour.

There is an important distinction between association (or, as we say in statistical terms, correlation) and causation. Researchers often find when they analyse their data, that two things seem to increase at the same time. Or maybe one thing apparently increases at the same time as another thing decreases, but they seem to change at the same time, so we say that they may be associated, or correlated (literally co-related). When we find what appear to be correlations, it is very tempting to conclude that one of them causes the other, and it is from here that we get the term causation. The temptation to think that two things are related is even greater if it already seems plausible that these things are related and/or if the research concerns a question which is highly emotive, such as whether something can save the lives of babies. Bevan *et al* (2019) pointed out that *"The retrospective and observational design of these studies makes it difficult to ascertain if the data are complete, or if the reduction is conclusively attributable to screening alone."*

I want to be very clear here. I am not saying that antibiotics don't help to prevent EOGBS disease at all. I am saying that, from a scientific perspective, the research that has been done to date unfortunately isn't good enough to tell us for sure whether giving antibiotics helps to reduce the rates of EOGBS disease or not. And if they do help, we can't tell how much difference they would make. Although antibiotics clearly cannot be anywhere near one hundred percent effective, because we still see babies with EOGBS disease born to women who were given them in labour. The only kind of research that can tell us whether two things are genuinely related, and thus whether antibiotics are truly effective, are randomised controlled trials. In such studies, all the other variables are held constant and the only thing that varies is the one being studied. Just as importantly, as I wrote above, nobody should know who is having the antibiotic and who is having the placebo. This is so we can ensure that people's preconceptions and other psychological aspects like the placebo effect aren't going to affect the care that women and babies receive and the assessments that are made; thus potentially bias the results.

As Ohlsson and Shah (2014) noted, the opportunity for good research in this area has all but been lost because the belief that antibiotics work to reduce EOGBS disease and should therefore be offered to women deemed to be at risk has become so accepted in practice. This belief is based on a number of assumptions which we cannot know to be true, and some evidence suggests that this belief is either incorrect or only partially correct. But let's look more closely at the evidence that we do have.

Eastwood *et al* (2014) looked at the situation in Ireland by means of a retrospective cohort study. While they clearly perceive antibiotics to be the best course of action, they also found (like Schrag *et al* 2002) that giving antibiotics in labour doesn't prevent all cases of EOGBS disease. This could be taken to mean that we need more robust research to understand better what is going on here. But often the best we can do is to look at how closely the guidelines are followed. Again, it is deemed unethical by some to have control groups of women not having antibiotics in order to see if prophylactic antibiotics work to reduce EOGBS disease in babies.

A number of studies have looked at whether giving antibiotics reduces the chance that a woman has GBS in or around her vagina, on the basis that this is considered a surrogate measure of antibiotic effectiveness. McNanley *et al* (2007) argue from their findings that penicillin reduces the rate of vaginal GBS carriage in women who have been found to be carrying GBS when tested. This study involved taking several swabs from the vaginas of 50 women who were receiving antibiotics during their labour and seeing if the colony count (or the number of GBS bacteria found on each successive swab) decreased. It did, and it seems plausible to think that the antibiotics contributed to this effect. However, this was a small study and, importantly, the researchers didn't study a control group of women who didn't have antibiotics. This means we don't know what would have happened to those women by comparison, or if antibiotics do help, how large the effect is. There may, as I mentioned earlier, be physiological processes in labour that help clear bacteria from the birth canal; we don't know and, unless we add a control group to such studies, we can't find out. It would also be useful to look at whether there is a difference depending on the environment in which a woman labours and gives birth. All of these things would be useful for women to be able to take into account when they make decisions about GBS.

What about measuring what happens to babies in the real world? Research by Turrentine *et al* (2013) showed that babies whose mothers had more than four hours of antibiotics in labour were less likely to be admitted to a special care unit and/or be diagnosed as having an infection than babies whose mothers had less than four hours of antibiotics in labour. This also seems to be suggestive of antibiotics being helpful. But in this case what we don't know is whether some of the decisions to admit these babies or diagnose and treat them for infection were made *because* the women had had fewer than four hours of antibiotics in labour. In this study, the diagnosis of sepsis was made on the basis of clinical signs of possible infection, which are arguably more subjective than the results of laboratory tests (although, as we saw earlier in the book, laboratory tests are not always accurate either). It might be that midwives or doctors were more concerned about these babies because they already perceived that it was important to treat women with more than four hours' worth of antibiotics. I certainly know many neonatologists who will recommend admitting and treating babies who are considered to be at risk for EOGBS disease as their mothers did not receive four hours' worth of antibiotics, for instance because labour was short.

It is hard to know how to summarise this area in a helpful way. There is a decent number of nationally-recognised studies and reports such as those by the CDC (2005, 2007, 2010b) and Schrag *et al* (2002) and data generated within these studies seem to show that the rate of EOGBS disease has come down since we started to screen and treat women. This suggests that antibiotics may work on a population basis. And the small trials show that antibiotics reduce the chance of babies becoming colonised with GBS. But it is important to remember that the same studies (Schrag *et al* 2002, Eastwood *et al* 2014) also show that antibiotics do not help in all cases and that none of these studies are of the quality needed to properly evaluate the effectiveness of antibiotic prophylaxis to prevent EOGBS disease. There is a great deal about this area that we do not know or fully understand.

Some people and organisations cite the results of some of the studies that I have discussed here as if they were unequivocal or undoubted fact, while others do not want to take the received view at face value, and this is why I have gone into some depth in this section. The fact that there aren't any decent randomised controlled trials in this area is a huge problem, and not just from the point of view of not wanting to over-intervene or medicalise women's labours, or because of concern about antibiotic resistance. If we think we already have the answer and thus see antibiotics as the only or best solution, we may miss other possible ways of dealing with the problem of EOGBS disease. These other ways might include knowledge that could help narrow down the number of babies who are 'at risk' and/or other forms of prophylaxis which could help to reduce that risk.

It is important to remember that doing nothing can be a reasonable option, especially when our knowledge in and of an area is questionable and antibiotic prophylaxis carries unwanted side effects. Even better is when this approach is accompanied by the careful attention of a trusted health professional who can help identify the babies who might need help in the early stage of a problem developing. It is distressing to many midwives and doctors that, in this age of universal recommendations and increasing guidelines and pathways restricting what we can and cannot do, the age-old skills of watching, waiting and acting skilfully and quickly when it is appropriate, are falling by the wayside.

If antibiotics, then which, and for how long?

I have already noted that different countries recommend different antibiotic regimes and that, no matter what the national recommendation, there is often regional or local variation, but I want to return to this question briefly to note that some antibiotics are more controversial than others. In most places, penicillin is the recommended prophylactic antibiotic.

As already mentioned, Co-amoxiclav isn't recommended because of an association with neonatal necrotising enterocolitis (a disease in which parts of the bowel are damaged, sometimes severely) in the ORACLE trial (Kenyon *et al* 2001a, 2001b).

Where women are allergic to penicillin, vancomycin is now recommended in the UK instead of clindamycin (Hughes *et al* 2017). This is also an option in other countries, such as New Zealand (Darlow *et al* 2015), but vancomycin is the subject of ongoing debate in medical journals. At least a decade ago, it was suggested that it was inappropriate to offer it as GBS prophylaxis because there is a perceived need to reserve it for women who really need it, rather than allowing resistance to this to develop with overuse (Pelaez *et al* 2009). Onwuchuruba *et al* (2014) later argued that it was not effective, but the principles on which this assertion was based were then challenged by Tse *et al* (2014), leading to a discussion about effectiveness versus resistance (Towers *et al* 2014). The existence of so much disagreement and debate in the medical literature is not very helpful to those who need to make decisions, although that is a function of the state of the science and not the fault of those involved in the debate.

In most areas, four hours' worth of antibiotics in labour is recommended. The origin of this appears to be partly traditional, but it has been widely adopted and is the basis of many of the research studies mentioned in this book.

The four-hour theory was briefly challenged by Barber *et al* (2008), who measured the level of antibiotic (penicillin) in the cord blood of babies born to women who had antibiotics in labour. They found that the levels of antibiotic in babies' blood increased over the first hour after the antibiotics were given to the baby's mother but then decreased after that.

However, more recent studies (Fairlie *et al* 2013, Turrentine *et al* 2013), have shown that the relationship between the antibiotic concentration in fluids such as blood and the effects of this on bacteria is rather more complex than thought (Turrentine 2014). A small study carried out in Montevideo, Uruguay showed that four hours' worth of antibiotics was needed in order to reduce the number of women testing positive for GBS carriage from 72% to 12% (Scasso *et al* 2014). Most practitioners continue to recommend at least four hours' worth of antibiotics. In many areas, if a woman does not receive adequate antibiotic coverage in labour then she may be asked to consent to her baby having intravenous antibiotics, which I shall discuss in chapter four.

The risks of antibiotics

On a global scale, antibiotic resistance is one of the most concerning risks of using antibiotics, especially when these are given to large numbers of woman and/or babies (Ledger 2006, Singleton 2007, Barcaite *et al* 2008, Joachim *et al* 2009, Lee *et al* 2010, Shore & Yudin 2012, Schrag & Verani 2013, Seale & Millar 2014, Hughes *et al* 2017). No-one wants to put babies at unnecessary risk, but there is an inherent irony here. The current screening and prophylaxis programme involves giving antibiotics to vast numbers of labouring women whose babies are deemed to be at higher risk of developing EOGBS disease (which is different from definitely having EOGBS disease). But a significant consequence of this programme may be that future generations will not have effective antibiotics for those babies who are diagnosed with actual disease. Furthermore, the babies whose mothers had antibiotics as a preventative measure during their birth may find that the same antibiotics aren't available to them as adults.

Another potentially enormous but unquantifiable risk relates to an area that we are only beginning to understand. I began this book by discussing the relationships between humans and bacteria. Scientists have started to use terms such as the human microbiome to discuss the range of micro-organisms that live on and within our bodies. Recent research shows that not only are many bacteria beneficial, but they need to be passed on to the baby during birth via its mother's vagina and have an important part to play in future health. This especially relates to the gut and digestion as well as many other areas of wellbeing (Turnbaugh *et al* 2007, Collado *et al* 2012). Scientists are concerned about the potential risks to antibiotic overuse both in general (Blaser 2011) and to the baby whose mother receives antibiotics in labour (Neu 2007, Broe *et al* 2014). This latter concern is supported by the research showing that one of the risks of caesarean birth is that these friendly bacteria do not get passed on, which can lead to problems in babies (Grönlund et al 1999, Blaser 2011, Azad et al 2016).

Problems arise because some antibiotics are not particularly selective, and many beneficial bacteria will be killed by them. This may have considerable but as yet unquantified knock-on effects in both women and babies (Stokholm et al 2013). Other antibiotics only kill certain types of bacteria, but all antibiotics can create changes in women's and babies' gut bacteria and faecal flora which can in turn cause gastro-intestinal problems. Some of these changes have been associated with an increased chance of postnatal yeast infection in women and babies (Dinsmoor et al 2005). We now have direct evidence that antibiotic prophylaxis for GBS changes the composition of a baby's microbiome, especially in breast-fed babies (Mazzola et al 2016) but we need more research into this area.

Anecdotally, a good many women report concern that both they and their babies have developed gut problems after they had agreed to have antibiotics in labour in an attempt to reduce the risk of EOGBS disease. A number of women and midwives have observed that, when a woman has had intrapartum antibiotics, a baby's cord has sometimes taken longer to fall off than expected. They have speculated that this may be due to a lack of normal bacteria. Possible associations like these need to be investigated.

Some of the more common but less severe side effects of antibiotics include disturbances to the digestive system including bloating, indigestion, feeling or being sick and/or having diarrhoea. NHS Choices (2014) estimate that around 1 in 10 people who take antibiotics experience these symptoms, and they estimate that around 1 in 15 people have a mild allergic reaction to antibiotics.

Intravenous antibiotics can occasionally cause severe allergic reactions in women (anaphylaxis), and such events can also pose a threat to the unborn baby (Dunn et al 1999, Jao, et al, 2006, Khan et al 2008, Berthier et al 2007, Chaudhuri *et al* 2008, Hughes *et al* 2017). This is a rare occurrence, and is estimated to occur in between 1 in 2000 and 1 in 10000 cases (NHS Choices 2014). The consequences of anaphylaxis can be very serious, which is one reason why many practitioners are reluctant to give intravenous antibiotics at home or in a community setting. Previous tolerance of any or a particular kind of antibiotic offers a degree of reassurance, but is never a guarantee of safety.

Antibiotics can affect a baby's immune system which in turn increases the chance of a baby being susceptible to other bacteria, e.g. ampicillin resistant *Enterobacteriaceae* (Edwards *et al* 2002, Bedford Russell & Murch 2006). Other potential effects on the baby's immune system were identified in studies by Glasgow *et al* (2007) and Ashkenazi-Hoffnung *et al* (2011). These researchers found that antibiotics given in labour increased the incidence of later bacterial infections in infants. Given the enormity of this problem, we have a scarcity of research and a review of this topic concluded that more work is needed (Seale & Miller 2014).

Increased rates of diseases such as asthma (Kozyrskyj *et al* 2011), allergy (Kozyrskyj *et al* 2011), childhood obesity (Ajslev *et al* 2011), eczema (Tsakok *et al* 2013) and obsessive compulsive disorder (Rees 2014) have all been associated with early exposure to antibiotics. There is currently a debate about whether early exposure to antibiotics is associated with type I diabetes. As with the discussion about the effectiveness of antibiotics above, I want to point out that most of the studies show association rather than causation; far more work is needed to confirm these concerns.

Some risks of antibiotic use noted in the literature relate only to when they are given during pregnancy. For instance, Andersen *et al* (2013) identified a possible link between antibiotic use in early pregnancy and miscarriage. Most women are not offered antibiotics for EOGBS disease prevention during pregnancy, however.

Finally, although this is not a direct risk of antibiotic usage *per se*, the choice of birth environment is an important factor. This can play a significant part in shaping the experience of the woman, baby and family. Women who are going to receive antibiotics in labour will generally (although not exclusively) be expected to give birth in hospital, and the risks of hospital birth can include a greater likelihood of having interventions and being exposed to 'unfamiliar' bacteria and other infective agents. These risks need to be considered in the context of the environment in which the woman will give birth and in which the baby will spend his or her first few days, and I will look at this more closely in the next section. In relation to the risks of antibiotics however, Eastwood *et al* (2014: 6) summed up the situation rather succinctly when they wrote that *"Ultimately, the long-term effects of antibiotic use in pregnancy on the infant are not known."*

GBS, antibiotics and place of birth

As I have now mentioned several times, one of the most significant downsides of GBS screening and prophylaxis is the way in which this can lead to limitations being placed on where a woman can give birth and on what care and treatment she can access. This is not just when women decide to decline antibiotic prophylaxis, but also when they decide to have antibiotics but are told that they can only have these under certain circumstances, for instance that they must attend hospital to give birth.

Let me say first that in most of the world, no-one can deny a woman the right to give birth at home if that is what she chooses. But if a woman who carries GBS wants to give birth at home and have intravenous antibiotics in labour, she may be told that this is not possible. There are a couple of reasons that health systems are reluctant to facilitate women having intravenous antibiotics at home. The first of these is that antibiotics are powerful drugs and allergic reactions (including anaphylaxis) are possible, so it is usually considered safer to give them in a setting with fast access to emergency facilities, drugs and equipment. In addition to this, local protocols generally dictate that drugs given intravenously need to be checked by two registered professionals (e.g. midwives) to reduce the chance of drug errors. Usually, especially in early labour, only one midwife is present at a woman's home until she nears the end of her labour. Sending a second midwife to check drugs would have implications for the care of other women, especially where there are staff shortages. This may vary between countries and will depend a little on the economics of health care provision in the local area.

I do know of situations where women have been given intravenous antibiotics at home, generally after a long discussion about the benefits and risks of this and the creation of an individualised plan of care, but these instances are relatively rare. It may be possible to negotiate this, but denying women intravenous antibiotics at home is not analogous to some of the other situations we encounter in which women are told they cannot make certain decisions. Serious concerns about giving intravenous antibiotics at home exist amongst community-based nurses and other professionals, and often patients will only be given intravenous antibiotics at home if they have previously and recently had the same dose of the same antibiotic in hospital. This is because it is then known that they haven't had an allergic reaction before, although even this is not a guarantee that they will not have a subsequent reaction. A severe, life-threatening allergic reaction to antibiotics requires a prompt, multi-disciplinary response and this is not possible outside of a hospital setting. Furthermore, many midwives do not carry the drugs needed to reverse a potential antibiotic-created emergency.

For all these reasons, while some women have been able to negotiate having antibiotics at home, it is not straightforward. I know of women wanting a home birth and intravenous antibiotics who went to the hospital in early labour, had antibiotics, and then went home.

If women who have decided to give birth in a midwifery-led birth centre are found to carry GBS, they may be told that they are no longer eligible to birth there. The most common reasons given for this are that the units do not have the facilities to deal with emergencies arising from the administration of antibiotics (as above) or that the units do not have the facilities or staff to care for or observe babies born to women who carry GBS. This presents a stark choice: the woman can either go to the hospital to give birth, or she can stay at home but (as above) she will be unlikely to get antibiotics if that is what she would want. However, this varies considerably in different areas, and it is best to find out what would happen locally, ideally before you decide whether or not to have screening. This is because it is not possible to 'un-know' your GBS carriage status and you may find that this knowledge changes professionals' perceptions of the available options (Wickham 2009).

Women who decide that they do not want to have antibiotics may also wish to consider the kind of care they would receive in different settings as a result of this choice. Again, women who have been found to carry GBS and who go to hospital may find that they are put under considerable pressure to accept antibiotics. If they decline antibiotics, as I will discuss in chapter four, they may find that they are under pressure to allow antibiotics to be given to their baby.

At the back of the book there is a section on resources that will help you identify resources and organisations which can give you more information about your rights.

Other possible forms of prophylaxis

A number of other types of prophylaxis have been used by women in an attempt to reduce GBS colonisation and/or the risk of EOGBS disease. Several of these could be said to come under the category of holistic therapies or home remedies. I make the distinction between reducing the chance of GBS colonisation and reducing the chance of EOGBS disease because I am well aware that a few women turn to other forms of prophylaxis not so much because they feel concerned about the risk of EOGBS disease in their babies, but because they find themselves in a situation where they feel unable to decline GBS testing and want to try and increase the chance that any GBS test that they are given will come back with a negative result. In one example, this was because a woman was told that a negative test was essential before she would be able to give birth in a midwifery-led unit. This is a shocking indictment of the maternity services, and a violation of human rights, because it totally goes against the ethos of women being able to make the decisions that are right for them.

Before we get into the substances that most people will imagine fall under this heading, such as garlic and chlorhexidine, I want to briefly mention that some women and caregivers have used or have at least considered using oral or intramuscular antibiotics rather than intravenous antibiotics.

We have very little knowledge about whether these are effective. A study by Gardner *et al* in 1979 showed oral antibiotics to be ineffective against GBS, and they have rarely been considered in relation to GBS since, although the RCOG (2012) also notes that they are variably absorbed in labour. These are prescription drugs in many countries, so by contrast to the alternative forms of prophylaxis that I am about to describe, which could be considered as home remedies, the situations in which women in high-income countries have taken oral or intramuscular antibiotics have usually been rather unusual ones involving the collaboration of a health care professional. Examples include situations where a woman wanted to give birth at home or had a severe needle phobia. In some low- and middle-income countries, it is possible to buy antibiotics over the counter.

Much of what we can say about the other possible types of GBS prophylaxis is similar to what I have said in relation to intravenous antibiotics. We don't have good enough research to know whether any of these alternative forms of prophylaxis are effective. As with antibiotics, some people swear by one or more of these but their knowledge isn't based on good randomised controlled trial evidence. Because the main focus of most of the alternative remedies (again, just as with antibiotics) is to clear the vagina and/or rectum of GBS bacteria, they may also disrupt the normal flora of the vagina. Alternative remedies may also carry a risk of local reaction or inflammation. Most of these remedies, however, do not carry the same risks of anaphylaxis or potential antibiotic resistance and I have not come across any association between the remedies discussed below and particular diseases, but I will discuss any specific concerns as I go through the other types of GBS prophylaxis which have been proposed.

Vaginal douching

Vaginal douching is an often-discussed form of prophylaxis for reducing vaginal GBS carriage. It has long been known that vaginal douching can cause a transient reduction of vaginal bacteria. Most of this effect is likely to be due to the simple act of washing the surface of the vagina, but the use of certain substances can further increase the reduction in bacterial numbers (Onderdonk et al 1992).

Generally, douching has downsides and midwives and doctors recommend that, unless there are signs of an infection, healthy women should trust the vagina to cleanse itself. However, douching has recently become more popular as a prophylactic intervention in certain situations in mainstream maternity care. Some surgeons are now advocating vaginal douching with an antiseptic solution prior to a caesarean, in the hope of reducing surgical site infections. A review of the research on this topic by Haas *et al* (2018) showed that *"...cleansing the vagina immediately before a cesarean delivery with either an iodine-based or chlorhexidine-based solution probably reduces the risk of infection of the uterus after a cesarean section. This benefit may be greater for women who have their cesarean delivery after their membranes have already ruptured or they are already in labor."* Few studies have looked at the effect of douching on vaginal bacteria. In a very small study that evaluated the effect of using douche preparations for various periods of time, Onderdonk *et al* (1992) found that douche preparations containing acetic acid or povidone-iodine were more effective at reducing bacterial count than when the same women used physiologic saline (salt water). By contrast, a Turkish study by Sakru *et al* (2006) who found that women who used soap for daily vaginal douching were actually more likely to have vaginal GBS than women who did not douche.

Chlorhexidine douching

The most commonly researched substance for vaginal douching for GBS is chlorhexidine: an antibacterial disinfectant. This is used for hand-washing and skin cleansing in many hospitals and is also an ingredient in many medical preparations, including mouthwashes, *Hibiscrub* and *Hibiclens*. Because its effect is transient (which means that, while it may temporarily remove bacteria from an area of the body, once it has worn off they will start to return again), most of the research has centred on looking at whether it can remove GBS bacteria during labour.

A Cochrane review of the use of vaginal chlorhexidine during labour to prevent EOGBS disease analysed the results of four studies which included 1125 term and preterm babies (Ohlsson *et al* 2014). As with antibiotics, some of the results showed that chlorhexidine might reduce GBS colonisation but there were concerns about the quality of the research and there is no evidence that chlorhexidine douching reduces EOGBS disease. Some women experienced mild side effects from chlorhexidine, such as stinging or local irritation. No side effects were reported in babies in the Cochrane review, but several other papers have discussed concerns that chlorhexidine can damage babies' skin, especially if they are preterm (Tamma *et al* 2010, Lashkari *et al* 2012, Paternoster *et al* 2017).

Some women choose to use chlorhexidine douching as an alternative to intravenous antibiotics despite the lack of evidence (Ross 2007). Chlorhexidine douching is sometimes combined with douching with other solutions such as vinegar and/or live yogurt (to replace 'good' bacteria), but I have not found any useful research on the effectiveness of this practice.

Before I move on, I want to share one of my favourite facts about GBS research, which I think it a really good illustration of the state of the science in this area. I noted in the paragraph above that data from 1125 babies were included in Cochrane-quality studies of chlorhexidine douching. Earlier in this chapter, when we looked at the Cochrane review of antibiotics for GBS prevention, we saw that data from 852 babies were included in Cochrane-quality studies of EOGBS disease prevention. More babies have been involved in good quality trials of chlorhexidine douching as an EOGBS prevention strategy than have been involved in good quality trials of intravenous antibiotics as an EOGBS disease prevention strategy.

Probiotics

Another theory is that taking oral probiotics or eating live yogurt might help reduce GBS carriage and thus the likelihood of a baby getting EOGBS disease. A couple of small pilot studies showed that, while the women who took probiotics had lower quantitative GBS colony counts, there wasn't a significant difference in vaginal GBS (Hanson *et al* 2014, Olsen *et al* 2018). In both studies, a significant number of women did not take the assigned probiotic, which reduces what we can learn from the findings. However, the women who did take the probiotics had lower GBS counts. Both teams concluded that we need larger, well-designed studies and that further research would be feasible and justified (Hanson *et al* 2014, Olsen *et al* 2018).

Aziz *et al* (2018) presented an overview of a randomised controlled trial (which at the time of publication had not yet been published in full) in which 251 women were randomised to take either oral probiotics or a placebo. The results showed that, *"No significant difference was found in GBS rectovaginal colonization at 35-37 weeks' gestation between probiotic supplementation vs. placebo (18.5% vs. 19.7%, p=0.87). Secondary outcomes were also not different between the two study arms."* (Aziz *et al* 2018). The information available thus far does not tell us how many of the women took the assigned probiotics. The authors of this study also call for further research testing different dosages and routes.

Probiotics can also be given locally via the vagina or rectum. A key reason that researchers think probiotic research should continue is because, unlike antibiotics, probiotics do not kill other beneficial bacteria but, as of now, we do not have any evidence of their effectiveness. It would be very interesting to look at prebiotics as well, but I have not found any studies on this topic in relation to GBS.

Garlic

A number of women have tried using garlic pessaries to reduce GBS carriage. Although there is some variation, the most commonly discussed approach is to peel and slightly crush a clove of garlic before inserting it into the vagina overnight. This is done for several nights in a row, and sometimes up until the baby is born. The garlic is removed (or it may fall out naturally) each morning. Anecdotally, side effects include itching or a slight burning sensation, which seems to be more likely when the garlic is fresher or when it is heavily crushed before insertion.

This practice has been described in the midwifery literature (Cohain 2004) but most of the discussion on this topic is anecdotal and speculative. Odent (2015) discussed a study by Cutler *et al* (2009) showing that a gel made from allicin, the active component of garlic, is effective against GBS. He states that such a gel reduces the main problems with the use of raw garlic; the difficulty of standardising the dose and tissue irritation. The next step in researching this would be a randomised controlled trial but, as Odent (2015) himself notes, there appears to be little interest in possible preventative strategies other than antibiotics.

Oral garlic is occasionally mentioned in relation to GBS, along with vitamin C and herbs such as echinacea, perhaps because they are used by some women as alternatives to antibiotics in other areas of health. However, we have already noted that oral antibiotics were long ago deemed ineffective (Gardner *et al* 1979). It may be that one reason oral forms of prophylaxis have not had as much attention in this area is the perception that it is more effective to use a preparation locally (in the vagina) in order to reduce GBS carriage. We do not have enough evidence on this area to know whether such forms of prophylaxis are effective.

Herbs

I know from talking to women, midwives, herbalists and birth workers that a number of herbal recipes are used around the world to attempt to prevent or eradicate GBS colonisation and/or EOGBS disease. Examples of herbs commonly used in this way include barberry, astralagus, burdock root, echinacea, horsetail and thyme. There are many different recipes and combinations, but I have not found any evidence on whether any herb, either alone or in combination with others, has any effect on GBS carriage or disease. This is probably to be expected given the dominance of the biomedical model and, as Odent (2015) noted, the difficulty of raising interest in alternatives, let alone funding.

Water birth

Many women want to use water during labour for reasons that have nothing to do with EOGBS disease prevention, and I will discuss this topic again in chapter four. Some people have realised that giving birth in water may in itself be a means of reducing the chance of a baby getting EOGBS disease. Although women who are carrying GBS or whose babies are seen to be at risk of getting EOGBS disease are sometimes advised against giving birth in water, Cohain (2010) pointed out that studies of water births show lower rates of EOGBS disease than are found in the general population. As these water birth studies did not set out to look specifically at issues relating to EOGBS disease and its prevention however, we ideally need more research which specifically considers this issue. It is important to note that some of the women whose babies are considered to be at risk in countries such as the UK may be advised against pool use for other reasons (for example, because they are in preterm labour) and not because of the EOGBS disease risk *per se*.

The only such study that I could find was carried out by Zanetti-Dällenbach *et al* (2007), and included 474 women who used water for labour and/or birth. Of those women, 213 stayed in the water to give birth, while 261 chose to get out before their baby was born. Before they got into the pool, the number of women carrying GBS in each group was similar. However, the babies who were born under water were significantly less likely to be colonised with GBS than the babies whose mothers laboured in water but gave birth on land. All other outcomes were similar between the groups. In order to know for sure whether water was an effective EOGBS disease prevention strategy, we would need to conduct a randomised controlled trial. However, it is not possible to use blinding as both the woman and her caregiver would know whether or not she was in the pool! A significant problem with carrying out such a study is that women in labour should be able to get in or out of a pool depending on what their feelings and needs are at the time and not as dictated by the randomisation method of a research study. As is happening with a number of other birth-related studies at the moment, we might not find many women who were happy to take part in such research.

If water birth does reduce the likelihood of a baby being colonised with GBS, there are a number of reasons why this might be the case, and several of these were discussed by Cohain (2010). The water may serve to dilute or wash off GBS bacteria. This was suggested by Zanetti-Dällenbach *et al* (2006), who found GBS in the water that GBS-carrier women had given birth in. Babies born under water are likely to stay skin-to-skin with their mothers, which may offer some protection and ensure early colonisation with the mother's bacteria. Babies born under water may also be less likely to be handled by other people and subjected to immediate interventions by comparison to land-born babies. We do need to consider, however, whether and how this might interfere with the normal colonisation of the baby with healthy bacteria, as with all of the other interventions designed to prevent GBS carriage, transfer and/or disease.

Caul birth

Anecdotally, some women and midwives have questioned whether being born in the caul (where the baby's waters do not release until or just after birth) is protective against EOGBS disease. While there is no systematic research into this (and likely will never be), this theory rests on the possibility that the intact membranes serve as a protective barrier. However, this is another example of a situation where any reduction in GBS bacteria may also mean a reduction in the bacteria that the baby is meant to pick up during and just after birth.

Arguably, being born in the caul does not really count as a prophylactic measure because it is not possible to avoid spontaneous release of the waters that surround the baby. It is not a case of being able to say *'I have decided to have my baby born in her caul'* in the same way that one can say, *'I have decided I want to use water during my labour.'* That's because, while it is entirely possible to decline artificial breaking of the waters, it's not possible to stop them from releasing spontaneously. But I am including this discussion here because some women are asked if they want to have their membranes artificially ruptured, usually as part of the process of induction of labour or in an attempt to speed labour up. It is not usually an effective way of speeding labour up, and it can have undesirable knock-on effects, but that is another book.

Women who are concerned about EOGBS disease, whatever their other decisions, may wish to ensure that their membranes (which form the baby's caul) stay intact for as long as physiologically possible and avoid other invasive interventions such as vaginal examinations, 'stretch and sweeps' and the use of fetal scalp electrodes.

Future possibilities and ongoing questions

Within medical circles, the main discussion as far as future forms of prophylaxis are concerned is that of a possible vaccine against GBS, not least because even proponents of the current screening and antibiotic prophylaxis regimens are aware that these have *"...inherent limitations"* (Schrag & Verani 2013: D20). The authors of a number of recent papers have cited the fact that research into a vaccine is in clinical development (Oster *et al* 2014, Sullivan & Soper 2015, Donders *et al* 2016, Madhi *et al* 2016, Ahmadzia & Heine 2014, Hughes *et al* 2017) and have noted that this would theoretically be cost-effective. However, this is still a good few years from becoming a reality in clinical practice, and there remain questions about whether a vaccine would be effective, safe and/or acceptable to women. One of the biggest potential controversies with a vaccine is that it would be offered to all women during (or possibly before) pregnancy, as we wouldn't know which women would be at risk of picking up GBS bacteria. These arguments are seen as less relevant by some of those who are concerned about growing levels of antibiotic resistance (Watts 2014).

Are there other avenues which could usefully be explored? This is purely speculative, but one thing that always strikes me about research into the majority of the possible forms of GBS prophylaxis, including antibiotics, chlorhexidine douching and water birth is that, while there is some evidence that all of these might help reduce the chance of a baby being colonised with GBS, we do not know enough about the possible relationship between a reduction in colonisation and a reduction in EOGBS disease. We do not know the exact mechanism by which EOGBS disease occurs, or what other factors may influence this. Some of the researchers who work on this topic have become so focused on eradicating the presence of GBS in the mothers of babies deemed to be at risk that we do not seem to be considering the many other important things that we don't yet know about in this area. Given how much our understanding of bacteria and their importance in our lives has moved on in the past few years, we may be missing the opportunity to reconsider this problem from a different angle and which may lead us to a better solution.

Research into several of the forms of prophylaxis which I have discussed in this chapter show that, while some of these prophylactic measures appear to reduce GBS carriage, they do not necessarily affect the occurrence of EOGBS disease in babies. This may be because we have not yet done good enough or large enough research studies. If we carried out a really good randomised controlled trial, we might show that one or more of these interventions are effective. But it might also be that carrying GBS is only one factor in developing EOGBS disease. It might even be that carrying GBS is a necessary starting point for EOGBS disease, but the actual disease is *triggered* by something else, which at the moment we don't even know to look for. But as long as there is a possibility that GBS disease has multiple causes, or is caused by something else in the presence of GBS bacteria, then the best thing that we can do for our current and future babies is to keep our minds open to other possibilities.

Some of these points have been raised by Odent (2015: 12), who asks some highly pertinent questions, as well as pointing out that, according to many theories, GBS is derived from a bovine ancestor and that *"...the emergence of GBS neonatal disease followed a major change in the collection of milk from farms, using bulk tanks rather than churns."* This may of course be coincidence rather than causation, but it is surprising that no-one has considered carrying out research to explore the questions which might arise from this theory. I also mentioned earlier that the antibodies that a woman herself carries may play a part.

In 2018, a fascinating paper was published in Scientific Reports. Hansen *et al* (2018) described their research which showed that bilirubin, a yellow substance involved in the breakdown of waste products in the human body, stops the growth of GBS bacteria. Bilirubin is the substance that makes a baby's skin look yellow when it has jaundice. Bilirubin is already known to be an antioxidant which is also beneficial when people have endotoxic shock; a consequence of serious infection. We are still in the early stage of our learning on this topic, but these researchers conclude that *"The data improve our understanding of the mechanisms modulating GBS survival in neonatal hyperbilirubinemia and suggest physiological jaundice may have an evolutionary role in protection against early-onset neonatal sepsis."* (Hansen *et al* 2018).

There is a fascinating corollary of this study. Its findings point to the possibility that the answer may not lie in the direction of giving man-made pharmaceutical products to women and babies or even using home remedies to try to remove GBS bacteria. Instead, there may be some value for some babies in stripping back unnecessary medical intervention such as early cord clamping, which deprives the baby of its blood and thus the bilirubin which Hansen *et al* (2018) found to be protective against early-onset sepsis. This would need to entail more respectful, woman-centred and physiologically-focused approaches to birth in healthy women and babies. That doesn't mean that it is the whole or only answer, though; we have large gaps in our knowledge.

There is a final approach, which many holistic midwives and doctors would frame as the employment of a watchful approach where we do not act unless there is a sign of a problem in the woman or baby. As one midwife noted, a key advantage of not acting to offer a specific form of prophylaxis – whether pharmaceutical, herbal or other in origin – is that, *"Whatever you actually do to lower colonisation of GBS or 'improve' vaginal health, the mother gets the message that her body is not good enough for the baby."*

The final alternative – at least as far as our current knowledge goes - is to screen and/or treat the baby rather than the mother. We tend to have this idea that, in pregnancy, it is OK for person A (the woman) to take on the risks of prevention in order to avoid person B (the baby) from experiencing harm. But is this always true or appropriate?

An obstetrician colleague pointed out that, *"We have a strong cultural belief that babies are fragile and incredibly precious (and don't get me wrong, I love my kids, but they did survive falling face first out of the pram often enough for me to know they are tough buggers), and that women will sacrifice anything to avoid harm coming to their baby. But once you remove the emotion from it, it makes more sense to jab the baby [rather than its mother] if they are deemed to be at risk."* I will look at this option at the beginning of the next chapter.

Our knowledge in this area is advancing and a number of different tests for infection and sepsis are currently being researched and brought into practice. It is my hope that, by the time I next update this book, we might have more knowledge which will provide another path for women who do not want to take antibiotics or to be vaccinated 'just in case.'

4. Wider issues and decisions

This chapter covers a number of wider issues related to decisions about GBS screening and prophylaxis. The first of these is what happens after the baby is born if there are concerns about GBS. I then go on to answer a number of frequently-asked questions about making decisions relating to the issues in this book.

Observing and treating newly born babies

It is not uncommon for people to ask why, if we are so worried about babies getting EOGBS disease, we don't wait for 'at risk' babies to come out and then give them antibiotics directly? Sometimes that does happen, and I will look at that in this chapter. The more usual answer to this question is that (a) research has shown that giving antibiotics to babies can do more harm than good (I will return to this below) and (b) EOGBS disease can occur so soon and escalate so quickly after a baby is born, that it is thought to be better to get the antibiotics into the baby's system sooner rather than later.

But not all babies who are deemed to be at risk have antibiotics given to their mother while she is in labour, for one or more reasons. Some women decide not to have antibiotics in labour, while some might plan to have antibiotics but give birth so quickly that there is not time for them to be given. Whatever the situation, where professionals feel that antibiotic coverage has not been adequate, some parents find that they are offered antibiotics and/or some kind of screening for their baby once it is born.

The screening offered to newborn babies ranges from observation of the baby's condition to blood tests looking for particular substances such as C-reactive protein (CRP), which indicates the presence of inflammation and is viewed as a marker for infection. In some areas of the world, a less invasive approach is used. For instance, the focus is placed more on observing a baby for signs of infection rather than immediately giving antibiotics. This is still deemed to be effective by many professionals and it saves time, cost and stress as well as reducing antibiotic prescription (Glackin *et al* 2015). However, conversations with midwives and doctors around the world continually demonstrate that, in practice, the range of what is offered in these circumstances is still incredibly varied, as the following examples illustrate:

"If the woman isn't given two doses of antibiotics prior to delivery, baby is recommended to have FBC (full blood count) and CRP at birth, four-hourly observations for 24 hours and then repeat CRP. If the CRP is greater than 7 at birth or greater than 15 at the 24-hour mark, the paediatricians recommend giving intravenous antibiotics to the baby for 48 hours."

"We don't do specific observations on babies if there have been 2 doses of antibiotics during labour. If less than 2 doses have been given then 4 hourly observations are done for 24 hours. If the baby is stable after 24 hours then s/he can go home."

"If there are 2 other risk factors such as prolonged rupture of membranes, maternal [raised] temperature in labour or prematurity then the babies get IV antibiotics for 48 hours too. I notice a lot of paediatricians use their own discretion here though and put more babies on antibiotics than they should."

"At our hospital [in Australia], *women aren't routinely screened for GBS, unlike in many hospitals. But the paediatricians do a heel prick test on all babies for CRP results at birth instead."*

"In the event of insufficient IV cover (this would be classed as less than 2 doses of antibiotics in labour or the second dose not being on board for at least 1 hour before the infant is born), then neonatal IV antibiotics are usually recommended."

Antibiotics do of course carry risks for newborn babies. We don't know enough about the potential harm to the baby when women are given antibiotics in labour, but antibiotics that are given directly to newly born babies have been associated with a number of unwanted outcomes including asthma, allergies, necrotizing enterocolitis and disseminated fungal infection; some of which can be fatal (Kozyrskyj *et al* 2011, Nash, *et al* 2014). They have also been linked with obesity (Ajslev *et al* 2011), psychiatric disorders (Rees 2014) and an increased chance of the baby being infected with other bacteria which have consequences just as severe as EOGBS disease (Edwards *et al* 2002, Bedford Russell & Murch 2006). In addition, as when given to adults, antibiotics can prevent or inhibit the growth of normal, healthy bacteria. This is a significant problem given what we know about the importance of babies becoming colonised with 'good' bacteria after birth.

Antibiotics can also be life-saving for babies who do need them, so women and their families will want to weigh up the risks and the benefits before making the decision that is right for them and their baby. Because of this, and because of the variation in practice in different areas, I would urge any woman who is considering bacteriological GBS screening or who may be deemed to have a risk factor to ask about the local guidelines, recommendations and usual practice as early as possible. As I noted in chapter one, the outcomes of babies who develop EOGBS disease vary according to whether a baby was born at full term or preterm. Some women prefer to take a 'wait and see' approach to a healthy baby, observing their baby for any signs of infection or other problems rather than giving antibiotics just in case.

Some of the midwives and doctors who I talked to shared their discomfort with the way in which women and their partners are sometimes spoken to about their decision to accept antibiotics or not. Because this is seen as a situation in which action must be taken soon after birth, the ideal approach is to be informed beforehand. Furthermore, where parents are keen to take an approach that deviates from the usual practice, it can be beneficial to begin this conversation ahead of time if that is possible. Below I share an example of a mother who chose to deviate from the usual practice and adapted what was recommended, but it would be unfair of me to imply that this is always an easy path, for some parents find themselves needing to negotiate with caregivers. One woman said:

"When I discovered the 'monitoring' at my hospital was likely to involve a doctor or midwife peering into the bassinet every few hours I felt I could do this myself and this confirmed my decision to stay at home. We woke up every couple of hours to take my daughter's temperature etc."

It is true that the observation element of monitoring a baby for signs of EOGBS disease is mostly a visual examination, and Cantoni *et al* (2013) argued from their research that standardised physical examination offered no advantage over a standard physical examination plus laboratory tests.

The tricky thing about observing babies for infection is that some of the signs of infection can also be seen in normal, healthy newborn babies. They can also appear as subtle changes rather than very obvious problems. For these reasons, and because infection can take hold and become very serious very quickly in newborn babies, a high index of suspicion is usually recommended, which means that it is considered better to err on the side of caution and check out something that may turn out to be benign than to be unconcerned about a sign that may be an indication of infection, even if it may also be something normal. Some of the signs of infection in babies are listed in the next section, but this list should not be considered a substitute for individualised care and advice from a midwife or doctor.

One final point that is worthy of note was raised by an obstetrician:

"Even though we know they aren't 100% effective, we only watch the babies that we decide (arbitrarily, based on poor data) to

be at increased risk. So does that mean that the ones who got antibiotics but go on to get sick may fall through the cracks?" This is a really important point, and one that should be shared with all parents, because even having every possible test and prophylaxis is no guarantee against EOGBS disease, and any parent who is concerned about their baby should seek help as quickly as possible, regardless of what testing or prophylaxis they have already received.

Signs of infection in babies

The following signs are the kind of things that professionals look for when judging whether a baby may have an infection. Any parent who is worried about a baby should always seek immediate midwifery or medical help, whether or not the baby has any of these signs.

Baby experiences respiratory distress: seems to be breathing faster than normal; is struggling to breathe; makes 'grunting' (high pitched squeaking noise when breathing out) or other unusual noises; stops breathing; takes long gaps between breaths.

Baby has a temperature of less than 36°C or more than 38°C; experiences temperature changes (either up or down); has poor peripheral perfusion (cold or pale hands or feet).

Baby experiences changes in heart rate or unexpectedly needs resuscitation.

Baby seems lethargic or floppy; their behaviour or responsiveness seems unusual.

Baby has feeding difficulties or refuses to feed; baby can't tolerate feed; experiences vomiting and/or has a distended abdomen.

Baby experiences seizure (fit).

Baby becomes jaundiced (yellow colouring of skin and/or whites of eyes) within 24 hours of birth.

Baby has signs of bleeding, which may manifest as bruises or unusual swelling, especially on the head.

Other signs of infection in babies include hypoglycaemia (low blood sugar), hypotension (low blood pressure), oxygen desaturation (lowered amount of oxygen being carried in the blood) and metabolic and/or respiratory acidosis. These are not things that can normally be checked without specialised knowledge and/or equipment.

GBS and breast milk

Sometimes, women ask whether feeding breast milk to babies is a risk factor for EOGBS disease. Although there have been a few incidences of late-onset GBS disease in babies whose mothers have then been found to have GBS in their breast milk (Wang *et al* 2007, Jones and Steele, 2012, Filleron *et al* 2014), most women who are carrying GBS do not carry this in their breast milk (Homer *et al* 2014). Even though some may do, the vast majority of breastfed babies are completely unaffected by GBS in breast milk (Le Doare & Kampmann 2014).

As Berardi *et al* (2014) discussed in a letter to a paediatric journal, this is a controversial situation for a number of reasons. It is hard to tell whether breast milk samples in some studies have been contaminated or whether the studies aren't of good quality. There are a number of routes by which GBS can be transmitted (including via health professionals and equipment), which means we can't be certain where a baby acquired GBS. As I mentioned at the beginning of the book, few people are willing to consider that health professionals, hospital furniture or equipment could be a source of EOGBS disease, instead placing all responsibility for this with the baby's mother by focusing only on vertical transmission. However, there is widespread agreement that late-onset GBS disease can be picked up from anyone who handles the baby, which means that breast milk is only one of a number of possible sources. For this and other reasons, most researchers stress that even rare instances of possible transmission via breast milk are uncertain and vastly outweighed by the positive benefits of breast milk to babies.

Even more recent research has focused on sugars in breast milk, known as human milk oligosaccharides or HMOs. These sugars affect the growth and cell biology of GBS and it is thought that they might confer some protection against GBS to breastfed babies (Ackerman *et al* 2017). Given that premature babies are at higher risk from EOGBS, this provides yet more evidence of the need to provide additional support to those women who want to breastfeed their premature baby.

GBS and the placenta

In recent years, the practice of consuming the placenta (also known as placentophagy) has become more popular, although it is still atypical rather than a common practice. Some women may consume part or all their placenta either raw (for instance blended in a smoothie) or cooked into a meal. There is a growing trend for birth workers to offer placental encapsulation, where the placenta is carefully treated, dried, ground and made into capsules. Some people think that there are benefits to consuming placenta, but there is little research on this so it remains a personal choice.

In 2016, the Centers for Disease Control (CDC) in the USA reported on a case where a baby had twice been admitted to a hospital for GBS disease. In both cases, the baby was successfully treated with antibiotics, but it was discovered during the process of trying to establish the source of the GBS that the woman had had her placenta encapsulated. When the encapsulated placenta was tested in a lab, it was found to contain GBS bacteria. Although the CDC report (CDC 2016) acknowledges that the baby could have been colonised by another method (e.g. from a family member), they share concerns about placental encapsulation, stating that:

"The placenta encapsulation process does not per se eradicate infectious pathogens; thus, placenta capsule ingestion should be avoided. In cases of maternal GBS colonization, chorioamnionitis, or early-onset neonatal GBS infection, ingestion of capsules containing contaminated placenta could heighten maternal colonization, thereby increasing an infant's risk for late-onset neonatal GBS infection." (CDC 2016)

Some placental encapsulation practitioners disagree with the CDC's claim, for a number of reasons. They argue that some methods of treating the placenta (for instance, steaming it at a high temperature for an appropriate amount of time) are enough to eradicate bacteria. They point out that the CDC report is based on just one case and is not the result of a robust and well-planned research study. That is true, although it is perfectly valid to report unusual cases in the literature. What is clear is that this area needs further investigation and research. States and health authorities do of course have a responsibility to investigate concerns. States and authorities also have a long history of trying to shut down community-based, women-led practices and there are a number of political elements to this issue, not least of which is the ever-present tendency to apportion blame to women's bodies (and, in this case, what is grown by them) rather than to look further afield.

Women's experiences of GBS screening and prophylaxis

We are coming to one of the most important parts of this book, which is a 'frequently asked question' section based upon questions and emails that have been asked of and sent to myself and to colleagues over the years by women themselves. Some of these women have allowed me to share their words in the final conclusion to this section; many more have allowed their questions and experiences to inform this book in a wider sense.

I hope I have shown throughout this book that there are many gaps in our knowledge in this area. We do not have good enough research about the screening and prophylaxis options that are currently offered to women, and there is little interest in exploring other paths even though some of these may be quite fruitful.

There is even less research into women's experiences of GBS screening and prophylaxis, although it is clear from the emails, comments and messages that I receive that many women are not happy with the current situation. Somewhat ironically, some women feel that we are overtreating and some women feel that we are undertreating. Sadly, some women feel that they are being bullied by others into having screening or accepting antibiotic prophylaxis that they do not want and that is not right for them or their baby. Others are concerned because they want more screening or prophylactic options than are offered in their area.

Quite understandably, some of those people whose babies have been lost to EOGBS disease are among those seeking to inform other women and families about the issue, and are some of the strongest proponents of universal screening and antibiotic prophylaxis. If you want to read published accounts of women's experiences of losing babies to EOGBS disease, you could look at the book *Mourning Sarah: a case for testing group B strep* (Huttlinger Vigour 2009) or the articles by Bodard-Williams (2013) or an anonymous mother (Anon 2001) who have all shared their stories.

The campaigns to promote GBS awareness are seen as incredibly positive by some people and as incredibly disempowering by others, as these women's words show:

"My 'journey' into maternity rights started when a huge yellow sticker (which made me feel a pariah at all appointments) was stuck onto my red book (maternity notes) without my consent. This was provided by the GBSS group and said 'Give Antibiotics when in labour.' When I questioned it, I was told I had no choice."

"I will always support the GBS campaign as I might have lost my baby if not for their information."

"I pretended I had lost the cover of my notes because I was so embarrassed by the sticker they put on them. It felt like they were singling me out as someone dirty. My midwife knew, and I think she agreed with me that it was horrible, but the assistant put it on before she even saw me so what could she do?"

"GBS is shrouded in a lot of confusion and misunderstanding - there are a lot of frightening sounding statistics used on sites that are clearly very biased towards hospital births with antibiotics for all."

"I'm glad to have the information. I'm the kind of person who wants to have every test I can get my hands on."

"Women don't realise that they have choices and options beyond what they are presented with by NHS staff. For example, I was told by a nice and well-meaning yet not knowledgeable on the subject community midwife that being GBS positive meant that I 'wouldn't get my lovely homebirth'. I ended up after a lot of research opting for the antibiotics in early labour and then going home again."

"It wasn't right for me. I wish I had been told that they would be testing my urine for this. I ended up having a nightmare last few weeks of pregnancy, feeling like I was battling to get my baby the birth I felt she deserved. Women's views should be respected. I wish there was an organisation that would do this and not just push antibiotics at you and try to scare you. They need to understand that having antibiotics is a scary option too, especially with what we know now about the benefits of bacteria."

These comments tend to reflect the ends of the spectrum of experience rather than the middle. That may be because it is the women, and others who feel the most strongly, who respond when people like myself invite comments about their experiences or about what kinds of issues of questions should be included on a book about this topic. So we also need research that approaches a wider spectrum of women and/or which talks to women who don't have prior experience, whether positive or negative.

One such research study was carried out in Ontario, Canada by Sharpe *et al* (2015). These researchers interviewed a small number of women who experienced GBS testing and antibiotic prophylaxis. In this kind of qualitative research, only small numbers of women are interviewed, because the researchers are looking to understand their individual experiences in depth. This can be incredibly useful, but it's always important to bear in mind that other women might feel differently and that not all women will be given the same range of screening and prophylactic options as the women in this study.

The results of this study are fascinating and will be useful for birth practitioners. Firstly, being found to carry GBS was *"...highly significant and frequently created dissonance"* (Sharpe *et al* 2015) for the women. Many women lacked knowledge of the issues and of their options.

"Prior to its administration, the test seemed straightforward and not very important for some women, and the treatment was seen as minimally invasive. One woman noted that the topic was

not discussed in a way that made her feel worried: *"The information...about the test itself and about the implications of getting antibiotics, it was all sort of conversational, and I was trying to piece it together in my head."* (Sharpe *et al* 2015). Such comments bring to question the balance between providing information and doing so without increasing women's anxiety.

Later however, *"The women in this study reacted to their positive diagnoses in a variety of ways. Some felt calm whereas others felt frustrated and annoyed. One woman felt alarmed by her diagnosis and noted, "I sort of went into like, outer space by myself at work for a while there. And I think, you know, they say when you tell people they have cancer, which is a terrible comparison, but they sort of stop listening after you get some kind of diagnosis." Another woman was less worried about the actual diagnosis, as she was annoyed with the "implications of it while being pregnant," such as possibly receiving IAP or needing to change her birth plans."* (Sharpe *et al* 2015)

In this study, women's experience of having intravenous antibiotics was also significant:

"The timing of the administration of IAP – and the tool itself – created anxiety and dissonance for the women involved in this study. In many people's minds, the IV is part of the medical construct and "may diminish [women's] labour and birth choices." The prospect of having an IV did not correspond to women's notions of midwifery care and created dissonance between what they thought "they were signing up for with midwifery care," as one woman put it, and what they found themselves experiencing. The IV made the experience feel "drastic" for one woman, who was challenged by the IV because she was "someone who is not used to medical intervention." With the IV, the woman who is GBS positive enters into a different reality and begins to compare her midwifery care with "medical care." (Sharpe *et al* 2015)

But one of the most positive outcomes of this research was the way in which the authors identified ways in which professionals can improve things, by considering language, information-giving and practice. I would like to end this chapter by drawing together a few ideas for midwifery, medical, doula and birth educator colleagues on this topic. First, it is important to avoid language which causes women to feel that they are dirty. I mentioned the use of positive language at the beginning of this book and the words that women shared with me for this chapter illustrate the value of this. Avoiding terms that are potentially offensive, disempowering or demeaning can go a long way towards helping women not to feel dirty as a result of finding out that they are carrying GBS bacteria.

Many women are dismayed to find that the level of risk that has been conveyed by a health professional or educator does not match the actual level of risk when they look at the figures. It is important to stress that EOGBS disease is very rare and that prophylaxis is not offered because it is likely but because the consequences can be severe for a small number of the babies who do develop it.

This is an area which is not at all cut-and-dried, and sometimes the most honest thing we can do in our communication is to say that none of the options are ideal and there is much that we do not know.

On a practical level, stickers or notes about a woman's GBS status should not be placed on the cover of her midwifery or medical notes without her permission. This has been raised by many women as a source of unnecessary distress. Some practitioners carry stickers or labels which can cover an unwanted GBS sticker that has previously been placed on a woman's notes without her consent.

Everyone involved in sharing information with women can try to ensure that options are presented as options and, perhaps most importantly of all, the focus should always be on respecting a woman's views and decisions, whether or not they reflect or contrast with those of the person offering information, education or care. It can be hard to switch around our language overnight, and this is especially true for those who have been educated within a patriarchal culture, but even small changes such as changing the word "give" to the word "offer" can go a long way.

5. Frequently asked questions

In this chapter, I briefly answer some of the questions which I have been asked and that have either not been directly addressed elsewhere in the book or are so common that I felt they were worth repeating here, for the sake of offering a quick reference guide.

Will I know ahead of time if my baby is deemed to be at risk of EOGBS disease?

The answer to this question depends on where you live. If you live in a country which recommends universal bacteriological screening during pregnancy and you decide to have this, you will know your GBS status ahead of time. The timing of this may vary for different women though, and there is lots of information on this in chapter two.

If you live in a country which uses risk-based screening, you may or may not know whether you or your baby is deemed to be at risk ahead of time. If, for instance, you have been coincidentally found to carry GBS on a test, you will know that you will be offered antibiotics in labour. But women who go into preterm labour will not know that this is going to happen ahead of time. Because of this, it can be reassuring to think through your options ahead of time and consider what your decision might be in different situations.

There is a full discussion of all the situations in which women in the UK may be offered antibiotics for GBS prophylaxis in chapter two. Women in other countries may wish to look up the relevant guidelines or ask their caregiver about this ahead of time.

If GBS testing isn't offered, can I request it?

You can always make a request, but this may or may not be granted, depending on where you live. Colleagues in New Zealand, for instance, tell me that it is not hard to get bacteriological testing there even though the national guidelines recommend risk-based screening, and they advise women to talk to their midwife or lead maternity carer.

In the UK, this may be more difficult, as the RCOG (Hughes *et al* 2017) now state that maternal request is not an indication for bacteriological screening. This does not mean it won't continue to be made available to women in some areas, but in other parts of the country the only way to have a bacteriological test in the absence of signs of infection is to undertake private testing.

How do I arrange a private test for GBS?

Some women in the UK or other countries which use a risk-based approach want to be tested for GBS even though this wouldn't normally be offered, so they either ask for this to be done through the maternity care system (which may or may not be successful, as already discussed) or they seek private testing. In the UK, at the time of writing a private GBS test costs between £40 and £65, depending on whether you purchase a postal test which you do yourself at home or whether you see someone who will carry out the test and report the results back to you. Your midwife or doctor may be able to point you to a local GBS testing facility should you wish to undertake private screening. It is also relatively easy to search for private laboratories on the internet.

Will the result of my private test be respected?

Usually, midwives and doctors are happy to accept the results of private screening tests, but it may be worth asking whether this will be the case before you pay for screening. Anecdotally, a couple of women have found that clinicians are more likely to accept a positive screening result from a private laboratory than a negative one.

Occasionally, women who want to be screened and/or treated for this encounter health professionals who do not seem to understand how important this is to them. If this happens to you, discuss your concerns with your midwife or doctor and/or talk to a midwifery manager or seek further support if you feel you are not getting what you need. You can get lots more information on decision-making and about your rights in *What's Right For Me?* (Wickham 2018a) and *Am I Allowed?* (Beech 2019).

Other than having antibiotics, are there things I can do to reduce the chance of my baby having GBS disease?

There's not much evidence on this, but avoiding artificial rupture of membranes (where the midwife or doctor breaks your waters rather than waiting for them to release naturally) and having as little intervention as possible (including vaginal examinations and stretch and sweeps) might help reduce the chance of your baby getting EOGBS disease, and/or reduce the amount of time in which your baby is exposed to GBS.

Given the recent research by Hansen *et al* (2018) that I discussed in chapter three, delaying cord clamping would seem to be a good idea. Some midwives and doctors believe that it can help to avoid interventions which break the baby's skin, such as the use of a fetal scalp electrode. But we do not have good evidence on this either, because no-one has researched it.

Having as much skin-to-skin contact between you and your baby as possible after the birth will help colonise the baby with your healthy bacteria. Breastfeeding will transfer antibodies to the baby, as well as offering a multitude of other benefits, including sugars which are protective against GBS (Ackerman *et al* 2017).

I have not been tested for GBS but have still been offered antibiotics. Why is this?

Unless there is some other reason that you have been offered antibiotics (and the best way to find this out is to ask the person who made this suggestion), this may be because you live in an area of the world where practitioners treat women whose GBS status is unknown as if they were carrying GBS. I know from midwives and doctors that this is a significant issue in some areas, but the exact details of such policies and practices vary.

In some regions that employ a universal screening approach, all women who have declined or not had testing are assumed to be carrying GBS. In other areas, the focus is on women who have specific risk factors. In some hospitals, for instance, women whose GBS status is unknown and whose waters have released for more than 18 hours without going into labour will be offered induction of labour and antibiotics. Similarly detailed guidelines exist in many areas, although there is often no evidence to suggest that the high level of intervention recommended will make any difference to the outcome.

If you find yourself in such a situation, it is worth asking some very detailed questions about why antibiotic prophylaxis is being recommended in your particular circumstances. This approach may or may not be in alignment with your own beliefs and goals for your birth. My book *What's Right For Me?* offers several ways to think about such decisions and suggestions of what kind of information to ask for when you find yourself in this kind of situation (Wickham 2018a).

Can I still have a water birth if I have GBS?

This will depend on where you choose to give birth. If you give birth at home, no-one can stop you using a pool or bath during labour and/or birth. If you give birth in a hospital or birth centre, regardless of anything to do with GBS or antibiotics, you cannot guarantee that you will be able to use the pool; a pool may not be empty or available or you may simply be told that you are not 'allowed' to use it.

But the answer to this question may also depend on whether or not you have decided to have intravenous antibiotics. There is no real reason why this should prevent most women using a pool, but some clinicians discourage women from using a birth pool or bath if they have an intravenous cannula in place. However, as I have described elsewhere, a small cannula can easily be removed and then re-sited later, if further doses of antibiotics are given. Or, if this really isn't possible, some midwives and doctors suggest covering it with a glove (like the midwives themselves wear) or plastic bag.

It may be that the midwife asks you to get out of the pool while the antibiotics are given. This is a safety precaution in case you have a severe reaction to the antibiotics.

Some women who have been found to carry GBS have been told that they are not eligible to use the pool in a birth centre or hospital. Unfortunately, there is not much that can be done about this situation because institutions do not have an obligation to provide facilities such as pools. It is worth discussing this ahead of time with your midwife or doctor. If using a pool is very important to you, you may wish to ask for a plan of care to be made which reflects your wishes or you might want to consider giving birth at home or in another birth centre where women who are carrying GBS are supported to give birth in water.

I want antibiotics in labour. How do I get them?

If you have a risk factor or have been found to carry GBS, it is not usually difficult to get antibiotics in labour. In fact, the opposite is true; it can be more difficult to decline antibiotics in labour. If you are concerned, talk to your midwife or doctor and ask to have a plan of care made before you go into labour. You may wish to discuss the different scenarios that might happen and what you would want to do in the case of each.

I'm planning a hospital birth. Will having antibiotics affect when I go to the hospital?

Women who know that they are carrying GBS and who decide ahead of time to have antibiotics when they go into labour are sometimes advised to go to hospital as soon as labour starts. This is so that there is the maximum possible chance that they will receive adequate antibiotic coverage before their baby is born. But there are downsides to going into hospital in early labour, including a higher chance of having certain interventions, including pain relief. As discussed elsewhere, antibiotics are not usually given until labour is established, but there is a balance to be struck here between wanting to make sure that labour is established (to prevent antibiotics being given unnecessarily) and wanting to ensure that antibiotics are started early enough to offer adequate coverage to the baby before she or he is born.

Somewhat paradoxically, some of the women who go in to hospital early (in some cases because they were advised to by one midwife or doctor) are sometimes then sent home again by another midwife or doctor without having had antibiotics, because they weren't deemed to be in established labour. This can be immensely frustrating.

I also know of more than one case where a woman who did not want to stay in hospital at that stage of her labour went in, had a dose of antibiotics, stayed long enough to ensure she was not having an allergic reaction, and then went home again. There are many possible permutations and situations. Overall, the best advice for women who are in this situation is to discuss, agree and document a plan of care ahead of time with their midwife.

I am worried that being screened for GBS will affect my planned home / birth centre birth?

Unfortunately, this is a very real concern. Some women have been told that they cannot give birth in a midwifery-led birth centre because they have been found to be carrying GBS, but no-one can deny you the right to give birth in your own home. You can decline screening if you do not want this and/or are concerned that this will affect your care. Despite having these rights, having a risk factor for GBS and/or being found to be positive for GBS can mean you come under pressure. In some situations and areas of the world, declining the test will mean that you are treated as if you are carrying GBS bacteria.

Again, it is worth talking to your midwife and finding out what the situation is locally. If you don't get the support you need, speak to a manager or seek support from one of the organisations that supports women and their birth rights. The resources section in the back of this book contains links to a number of further resources which may be of use.

What if I don't want to be screened for GBS?

Screening is not compulsory and you can decline any screening test that you do not want to have. However, it is important to remember that GBS screening is not always presented as such, and that GBS may be found anytime a vaginal or perianal swab or urine sample is tested. This does not apply to urine tests that are done with urine dipsticks; GBS tests can only be carried out when a urine sample is collected in a pot and sent to a laboratory.

If you are offered any test, you should always ask what it is for, why the midwife or doctor is offering it and what will happen when the results come back. If you are concerned about the implications of such testing for your options in labour, you should discuss this with the midwife or doctor before agreeing to the test.

You always have the right to decline having a test, to ask for a second opinion, to take time to think about it or to speak to a midwifery manager, consultant midwife (if available) or a birthing rights organisation for more support.

My GBS test was positive or I have a risk factor but I don't want antibiotics in labour?

You do not have to consent to anything that you do not want to have. Your midwife or doctor may be (or may feel) obliged to offer or recommend antibiotics and to ensure that you have full information about what is being suggested, but it is your body, your baby and your decision.

If a woman who is known to be carrying GBS or has known risk factors wishes to decline antibiotics when she is in labour, it is not uncommon for senior staff to get involved. This can seem punitive, but it is done to ensure that the woman has all the relevant information. It can sometimes be a good way for women to ensure that they will get what they want when they are in labour because, in many countries, professionals have an obligation to ensure that the woman has appropriate information and support; ideally, this will be an opportunity for the woman and her caregiver to develop a plan of care together that will meet the woman's needs.

Where a woman decides to decline antibiotics and make an alternative plan, a common suggestion is that the baby will be observed in the hospital every four hours for the first 24 hours, with further discussion about antibiotics for the baby if she or he shows any signs of infection. Some women who have planned a home birth and do not want antibiotics have negotiated a plan whereby they do this and a midwife visits a couple of times within the first 24 hours and closely observes the baby for any signs of infection. In this situation, the woman observes the baby in between the midwife's visits, following good instruction from the midwife regarding signs of infection and details of when to call for help clearly written down.

Remember that you do not have to agree to anything that you do not want to. If you feel that there is a chance that you will be put under undue pressure, set up whatever support you can ahead of time. This might include an independent midwife, a doula, partner, friend or family member who has read up on the topic and is willing and able to support and advocate for you if required.

Many organisations and people exist to support women who need support in exercising their rights during pregnancy and childbirth and you can find out more in the resources section at the back of this book.

Can I have a home birth if I am carrying GBS and/or have a risk factor?

In most areas of the world, no test result or risk factor can prevent you from having a home birth. You are not obliged to go to hospital or anywhere else to give birth, and you are not obliged to consent to anything that you do not want to consent to.

Your body, your baby, your decision.

That doesn't mean that it's not a good idea to consider the information about any possible pros and cons that you may receive from a trusted birth professional though, as they may have access to information and experience that you don't. This is especially the case if you are told that you or your baby have a particular risk factor.

If you decide you want to birth at home then, depending on where you live and on the quality of the local service, you may have no problem. However, you may find that pressure is put upon you to go into hospital or (if you are in a country where you are entitled to state-funded midwifery care) you may be told that a midwife may not be able to attend your birth. If you are in the UK, the brilliant book *Am I Allowed?* (Beech 2019) contains more information on this. Women in other countries may be able to find out more through home birth groups, midwives or organisations in their country (see the resources section for links that may help with this).

If you want to have intravenous antibiotics however, you may find that you are told that it is not possible to have these at home. As an expert in human rights in maternity care summarised for this book: *"A health care provider has no obligation to provide an intervention that they don't consider to be in a patient's best interest. In the case of intravenous antibiotics, the small risk of anaphylaxis may be considered 'a risk too far' by a doctor or midwife."*

Can I get alternative forms of prophylaxis from a midwife?

This depends very much on where you live, who your midwife is and what constraints they face. Some midwives and doctors are able to practice more autonomously than others. As things currently stand in the UK, for instance, it is unusual to get support for or information about alternative remedies from midwives or doctors who work in the NHS or other systems of maternity care. This is because their recommendations are expected to be in line with guidelines approved by their employer and these alternative or home remedies are not recommended. But some midwives are able to work more autonomously, both in the UK and elsewhere.

Women in more medicalised countries may be less likely to find people who are able to support them within the maternity care system, but an independent practitioner may be able to help you. Many women look for information on alternatives elsewhere, including on the internet, but please remember that such information is of hugely variable quality, there isn't evidence to support their effectiveness and so-called 'natural' remedies can have unwanted side effects and remove beneficial bacteria as well as GBS.

What if I can't get the care I want?

Every hospital and maternity system should have a complaints process and someone that you can speak to if you are not getting your needs met. In some countries, it is relatively simple to change provider, but in others it is not as straightforward. You could contact the head of midwifery, the maternity department manager or a consultant midwife. The resources section offers links to ways to find organisations that may also be able to help.

I declined antibiotics but have now been told that my baby must have them – can I decline?

This can be a tricky situation, because women and their partners can find themselves under a great deal of pressure to have antibiotics given to their baby, and some women have even been threatened with legal action and/or being reported to Social Services or a child welfare authority. In most countries, this is not a Social Services issue, and reporting is unlikely to lead anywhere. Nevertheless, the process can be distressing and time consuming at a stage where families want to be together without too much pressure and outside interruption.

The important thing to understand in this situation is that, while all decisions rest with the woman while the baby is unborn, a newborn baby is a person in their own right who has rights of their own. Doctors who look after newborn babies have a legal duty of care to those babies. If a doctor feels that parents are potentially compromising a baby's health and putting her or him at risk, they do have a degree of legal power. As a fact sheet on consent (in a UK setting) explains:

"Consent for any medical treatment or procedure, including the administration of a drug, must be sought from a person with 'parental responsibility' for the baby. This always includes the baby's mother, but the baby's father has parental responsibility only if certain criteria are met. You can find a summary of parental responsibility on the NHS Choices website.

If parents refuse treatment for their child, healthcare professionals should respect their decision. In some circumstances, including if parents disagree about treatment, healthcare professionals may approach the High Court for an order declaring that treatment is in a child's best interests and should be carried out." (Birthrights 2013: 4).

Some people feel that the key is to ensure that you do not give the doctor or other staff any reason to think that you are being reckless or unreasonable. It can help to stay calm, be clear about your concerns and engage in a two-way conversation. This demonstrates that you are open to discussion and respectful of the staff's expertise (even if this is not how you feel). You may wish to explain your understanding that EOGBS disease is rare and that you are more concerned about the long-term risks of antibiotics to your baby's health, which are relatively unknown.

"We explained [to the] neonatologist that we were concerned about possible side effects, later antibiotic resistance, gut problems and other negative consequences of antibiotics. I think it helped to use the medical terms, and definitely it helped to be calm and let them know that we really understood the risks of GBS. We said we were happy for our baby to be observed and that we wouldn't oppose antibiotics if there were actual signs of infection, and I offered to sign a page in my notes where we wrote this plan down, but that I didn't want him to have antibiotics just in case."

You could try contacting a midwifery/maternity manager or a consultant midwife or similar person for support, especially if they have been helpful to you in the past, but their role is a little different in this situation. In the UK and some other countries, you are more likely to encounter the 'safeguarding' midwife, whose role is more about the protection of babies. Some women engage an independent midwife, doula or friend to support them and there are, again, groups who will support women in this situation. You can find out how to access more information on this area in the resources section.

In conclusion

I always think it is important to try to give a balanced view of these very tricky and complex issues. I haven't urged women to take every test possible and to agree to intravenous antibiotics during labour, because that is not the only reasonable decision to make, particularly given the rarity of EOGBS disease. However, I hope I haven't made my reader think that GBS is something to dismiss, or that having antibiotics is always inadvisable. As is so often the case in decisions relating to pregnancy and birth, the evidence is unclear and often lacking, the options can weigh heavily and no decision comes with a guarantee.

Rarely, GBS can cause a life-threatening and sometimes fatal disease, but the vast majority of women who carry it won't be affected, and neither will their babies. Accepting prophylactic antibiotics does not offer any guarantee, and screening and prophylaxis may limit a woman's options and confer other risks. But the fact that we can't always prevent EOGBS disease and that our efforts to prevent EOGBS disease can cause other problems doesn't make it less of a life-threatening disease to those few babies who develop it.

Ultimately, it is up to you whether you have screening to see if you are carrying GBS bacteria. If you are found to be carrying this, or if you are told you have a risk factor, it is up to you to decide whether or not to have intravenous antibiotics in labour. If you decline these (or if they aren't deemed to have been adequate) but staff are worried about your baby, it is usually up to you to decide whether or not you want your healthy baby to have antibiotics 'just in case'.

Whatever you decide, I hope this book has helped you to better understand the issues relating to GBS bacteria and EOGBS disease and given you information to help you make the decisions that are right for you.

If you have enjoyed this book and found it useful, please leave a review at your favourite book retailer – it really helps highlight it to others who might need it!

To see more of Sara's work:

Visit me at www.sarawickham.com

Sign up for my free monthly newsletter and get information on new books, courses and projects at www.tinyurl.com/saranews

Hang out with me on Instagram, I'm @drsarawickham

I'm also on Facebook at www.facebook.com/saramidwife

References

Åberg E, Ottosson A, Granlund M *et al* (2018). Harbouring group B streptococci in a neonatal intensive care unit led to an outbreak among preterm infants. Acta Paediatrica 108(1):58-61.

Ackerman DL, Doster RS, Weitkamp J-H *et al* (2017). Human Milk Oligosaccharides Exhibit Antimicrobial and Antibiofilm Properties against Group B Streptococcus. ACS Infectious Diseases 3:595-605.

AAP (1992). American Academy of Pediatrics Committee on Infectious Diseases and Committee on Fetus and Newborn. Guidelines for prevention of group B streptococcal infection by chemoprophylaxis. Pediatrics 90: 775-8.

Abdelazim IA (2013). Intrapartum polymerase chain reaction for detection of group B streptococcus colonisation. Australian and New Zealand Journal of Obstetrics and Gynaecology 53(3): 236-242.

ACOG (1992). Committee on Technical Bulletins of the American College of Obstetricians and Gynecologists Group B streptococcal infections in pregnancy. ACOG Technical Bulletin 170:1-5.

Adriaenssens N, Coenen S & Versporten A (2011). European Surveillance of Antimicrobial Consumption (ESAC): outpatient antibiotic use in Europe (1997–2009). Journal of Antimicrobial Chemotherapy 66(Suppl 6): vi3–12.

Ahmadzia HK & Heine RP (2014). Diagnosis and management of group B streptococcus in pregnancy. Obstetrics and Gynecology Clinics of North America 41: 629-47.

Ajslev TA, Andersen CS and Gamborg M (2011). Childhood overweight after establishment of the gut microbiota: the role of delivery mode, pre-pregnancy weight and early administration of antibiotics. International Journal of Obesity 35: 522–9.

Andersen JT, Petersen M & Jimenez-Solem E (2013). Clarithromycin in early pregnancy and the risk of miscarriage and malformation. PLoS ONE https://doi.org/10.1371/journal.pone.0053327

Anon (2001). Caroline's Story. AIMS Journal 13(3): 15-17.

Anonymous Author (2017). Informed consent in theatre. The Practising Midwife 29(11): 47-50.

Ashkenazi-Hoffnung L, Melamed N & Ben-Haroush A (2011). The association of intrapartum antibiotic exposure with the incidence and antibiotic resistance of infantile late-onset serious bacterial infections. Clinical Pediatrics 50(9): 827-33.

Azad MB, Konya T, Persaud RR et al (2016). Impact of maternal intrapartum antibiotics, method of birth and breastfeeding on gut microbiota during the first year of life: a prospective cohort study. British Journal of Obstetrics & Gynaecology 123(6):983-93.

Aziz N, Spiegel A, Bentley J et al (2018). Evaluation of probiotic oral supplementation effects on group B streptococcus rectovaginal colonization in pregnant women: a randomized double-blind placebo-controlled trial. American Journal of Obstetrics and Gynecology 219(6): 638.

Baker CJ & Barrett FF (1973). Transmission of group B streptococci among parturient women and their neonates. Journal of Pediatrics 83: 919-25.

Barber EL, Zhao G & Buhimschi IA (2008). Duration of intrapartum prophylaxis and concentration of penicillin G in fetal serum at delivery. Obstetrics and Gynecology 112(2): 265-270.

Barcaite E, Bartusevicius A. & Tameliene R (2008). Prevalence of maternal group B streptococcal colonisation in European countries. Acta Obstetricia et Gynecologica Scandinavica 87(3): 260-71.

Barcaite E Bartusevicius A & Tameliene R (2012). Group B streptococcus and Escherichia coli colonization in pregnant women and neonates in Lithuania. International Journal of Gynecology and Obstetrics 117(1): 69-73.

Bedford Russell AR & Murch S (2006). Could peripartum antibiotics have delayed health consequences for the infant? British Journal of Obstetrics and Gynaecology 113(7): 758-765.

Beech BAL (2019). Am I Allowed. Second edition. Birth Practice and Politics Forum: forthcoming.

Berardi A, Di Fazzio G, Gavioli S *et al* (2011). Universal antenatal screening for group B streptococcus in Emilia-Romagna. Journal of Medical Screening 18(2): 60-64.

Berardi A, Rossi C & Guidotti I (2014). Group B streptococci in milk and neonatal colonisation. Archives of Disease in Childhood 99(4): 395.

Berthier A, Senthiles L & Hamou L (2007). Antibiotics at term. Questions about five allergic accidents. Gynécologie, Obstétrique & Fertilité 35: 464–72.

Bevan D, White A, Marshall J *et al* (2019). Modelling the effect of the introduction of antenatal screening for group B *Streptococcus* (GBS) carriage in the UK. BMJ Open doi: 10.1136/bmjopen-2018-024324

Bienenfeld S, Rodriguez-Riesco LG, Heyborne KD *et al* (2016). Avoiding Inadequate Intrapartum Antibiotic Prophylaxis for Group B Streptococci. Obstetrics and Gynecology 128(3): 598-603.

Birthrights, 2013. Consenting to treatment. Available at: http://www.birthrights.org.uk/library/factsheets/Consenting-to-Treatment.pdf

Blaser M (2011). Antibiotic overuse: Stop the killing of beneficial bacteria. Nature 476: 393–94.

Bodard-Williams C (2013). Group B strep infection: a mother's perspective. The Practising Midwife 16(2): 17-19.

Braye K, Xu F, Ferguson J *et al* (2017). Is exposing around a third of our birthing population to intrapartum antibiotic prophylaxis (IAP) for prevention of Early Onset Group B *Streptococcal* infection doing more harm than good? Women and Birth 30(Suppl): 24.

143

Briody VA, Albright CM, Has P *et al* (2016). Use of Cefazolin for group B streptococci prophylaxis in women reporting a penicillin allergy without anaphylaxis. Obstetrics and Gynecology 127(3): 577-83.

Broe A, Pottegård A & Lamont RF (2014). Increasing use of antibiotics in pregnancy during the period 2000–2010: prevalence, timing, category, and demographics. British Journal of Obstetrics and Gynaecology 121(8): 988-96.

Cabrera-Rubio R, Collado MC, Laitinen K *et al* (2012). The human milk microbiome changes over lactation and is shaped by maternal weight and mode of delivery. The American Journal of Clinical Nutrition 96: 544-551.

Cantoni L, Ronfani L. & Da Riol R (2013). Physical examination instead of laboratory tests for most infants born to mothers colonized with group B Streptococcus: support for the Centers for Disease Control and Prevention's 2010 recommendations. Journal of Pediatrics 163(2): 568-573.

Carstensen H, Christensen KK & Grennert L (1988). Early-onset neonatal group B streptococcal septicaemia in siblings. Journal of Infection 17(3): 201-4.

Centers for Disease Control and Prevention (2005). Early-onset and late-onset neonatal group B streptococcal disease-United States, 1996-2004. Morbidity and Mortality Weekly Report, 54(47): 1205-8.

Centers for Disease Control and Prevention (2007). Perinatal group B streptococcal disease after universal screening recommendations-United States, 2003-2005. Morbidity and Mortality Weekly Report, 56: 701-5.

Centers for Disease Control and Prevention (2010a). ABCs report: Group B streptococcus.

Centers for Disease Control and Prevention (2010b). Prevention of perinatal group B streptococcal disease: revised guidelines from CDC, 2010. Morbidity & Mortality Weekly Report 2010: 59 (RR-10).

144

Centers for Disease Control and Prevention (2012). Active Bacterial Core Surveillance Report, Emerging Infections Program Network, Group B Streptococcus.

Centers for Disease Control and Prevention (2016). Notes from the Field: Late-onset infant group B streptococcus infection associated with maternal consumption of capsules containing dehydrated placenta – Oregon 66(25):677-78.

Chan G, Modak J & Mahmud A (2013). Maternal and neonatal colonization in Bangladesh: prevalences, etiologies and risk factors. Journal of Perinatology 33(12): 971-76.

Chan WS, Chua SC, Gidding HF *et al* (2014). Rapid identification of group B streptococcus carriage by PCR to assist in the management of women with prelabour rupture of membranes in term pregnancy. Australia and New Zealand Journal of Obstetrics and Gynaecology 54(2): 138-45.

Chaudhuri K, Gonzales J & Jesurun CA (2008). Anaphylactic shock in pregnancy: a case study and review of the literature. International Journal of Obstetric Anesthesia 17: 350-57.

Cohain JS (2004). GBS, pregnancy and garlic: be a part of the solution. Midwifery Today 72: 24-25.

Cohain JS (2010). Newborn group B strep infection: Top 10 reasons not to culture at 36 weeks. Midwifery Today 94: 15.

Colbourn T & Gilbert R (2007). An overview of the natural history of early onset group B streptococcal disease in the UK. Early Human Development 18(3): 149-56.

Collado MC, Cernada M & Baüerl C (2012). Microbial ecology and host-microbiota interactions during early life stages. Gut Microbes 3(4): 352-65.

Cutler RR, Odent M, Hajj-Ahmad H *et al* (2009). In vitro activity of an aqueous allicin extract and a novel allicin topical gel formulation against Lancefield group B streptococci. Journal of Antimicrobial Chemotherapy 63(1): 151-54.

Dadvand P, Basagana X & Figueras F (2011). Climate and group B streptococci colonisation during pregnancy: present implications and future concerns. British Journal of Obstetrics and Gynaecology 118(11): 1396-1400.

Daniels J, Gray J & Pattison H (2009). Rapid testing for group B streptococcus during labour: a test accuracy study with evaluation of acceptability and cost-effectiveness. Health Technology Assessment 13(42): 178.

Darlow B, Campbell N, Austin N *et al* (2015). The prevention of early-onset neonatal group B streptococcus infection: New Zealand Consensus Guidelines 2014. New Zealand Medical Journal 128(1425): 69-76.

Davis-Floyd, Robbie E (1992). Birth as an American Rite of Passage. Berkeley, University of California Press.

De Luca C, Buono N, Santillo V *et al* (2015). Screening and management of maternal colonization with Streptococcus agalactiae: an Italian cohort study. Journal of Maternal Fetal and Neonatal Medicine 29(6):911-5.

de Steenwinkel F, Tak H & Muller A (2008). Low carriage rate of group B streptococcus in pregnant women in Maputo, Mozambique. Tropical Medicine and International Health 13(3): 427-29.

Dillon HC, Khare S & Gray BM (1987). Group B streptococcal carriage and disease: a 6-year prospective study. Journal of Pediatrics 110: 31-6.

Dinsmoor MJ, Viloria R & Leif L (2005). Use of intrapartum antibiotics and the incidence of postnatal maternal and neonatal yeast infections. Obstetrics & Gynecology 106: 19-22.

Donders GGG, Halperin SA, Devlieger R *et al* (2016). Maternal immunization with an investigational trivalent group B streptococcal vaccine: a randomized controlled trial. Obstetrics & Gynecology 127(2): 213-21.

Dunn AB, Blomquist J & Khouzami V (1999). Anaphylaxis in labor secondary to prophylaxis against group B streptococcus: a case report. Journal of Reproductive Medicine 44(4): 381-84.

Eastwood KA, Craig S & Sidhu H (2014). Prevention of early-onset Group B Streptococcal disease – the Northern Ireland experience. British Journal of Obstetrics and Gynaecology 122(3):361-7.

Edwards NP (2005). Birthing Autonomy: Women's Experiences of Planning Home Births. Oxford, Routledge.

Edwards RK, Tang Y, Raglan GB *et al* (2015). Survey of American Obstetricians Regarding Group B Streptococcus: Opinions and Practice Patterns. American Journal of Obstetrics and Gynecology 213(2): 229.e1–229.e7.

Edwards RK, Clark P & Sistrom CL (2002). Intrapartum antibiotic prophylaxis 1: Relative effects of recommended antibiotics on gram-negative pathogens. Obstetrics & Gynecology 100: 534-9.

El Helali N, Giovangrandi Y & Guyot K (2012). Cost and effectiveness of intrapartum group B streptococcus polymerase chain reaction screening for term deliveries. Obstetrics & Gynecology 119(4): 822-29.

Fairlie T, Zell ER & Schrag S (2013). Effectiveness of intrapartum antibiotic prophylaxis for prevention of early-onset group B streptococcal disease. Obstetrics & Gynecology 121: 570–77.

Faro JP, Bishop K & Riddle G (2013). Accuracy of an accelerated, culture-based assay for detection of group B streptococcus. Infectious Diseases in Obstetrics & Gynecology 2015: 367935.

Filleron A, Lombard F & Jacquot A (2014). Group B streptococci in milk and late neonatal infections: an analysis of cases in the literature. Archives of Disease in Childhood, Fetal and Neonatal Edition 99(1): F41-F47.

Florindo C, Damiao V & Lima J (2014). Accuracy of prenatal culture in predicting intrapartum group B streptococcus colonization status. Journal of Maternal-Fetal & Neonatal Medicine 27(6): 640-42.

Foxman B, Gillespie BW, Manning SD *et al* (2007). Risk factors for group B streptococcal colonization: potential for different transmission systems by capsular type. Annals of Epidemiology 17(11): 854-62.

Foxman B, de Azevedo CLB, Buxton M *et al* (2008). Acquisition and Transmission of Group B Streptococcus during Pregnancy. The Journal of Infectious Diseases 198(9): 1375-78.

Gardner SE, Yow MD & Leeds LJ (1979). Failure of penicillin to eradicate group B streptococcal colonization in the pregnant woman. A couple study. American Journal of Obstetrics and Gynecology 135: 1062–65.

Garland SM & Kelly N (1995). A study of Group B Streptococcus in Brisbane; the epidemiology, detection by PCR assay and serovar prevalence. Medical Journal Australia 162: 413-17.

Glackin S, Miletin I, Deasy AM *et al* (2015). A less invasive approach to screening for early onset neonatal GBS. Irish Medical Journal 108(3): 81-3.

Glasgow TS, Speakman M & Firth S (2007). Clinical and economic outcomes for term infants associated with increasing administration of antibiotics to their mothers. Paediatric and Perinatal Epidemiology 21(4): 338-46.

Grimwood K, Stone PR & Gosling IA (2002). Late antenatal carriage of group B Streptococcus by New Zealand women. Australian and New Zealand Journal of Obstetrics and Gynaecology 42(2): 182-86.

Grönlund MM, Lehtonen OP & Eerola E (1999). Fecal microflora in healthy infants born by different methods of delivery: permanent changes in intestinal flora after cesarean delivery. Journal of Pediatric Gastroenterology and Nutrition 28(1): 19-25.

Haas DM, Morgan S, Contreras K *et al* (2018). Vaginal preparation with antiseptic solution before cesarean section for preventing postoperative infections. Cochrane Database of Systematic Reviews Issue 7. Art. No.: CD007892.

Håkansson S & Källén K (2006). Impact and risk factors for early-onset group B streptococcal morbidity: analysis of a national, population-based cohort in Sweden 1997-2001. British Journal of Obstetrics and Gynaecology 113: 1452-58.

Håkansson S, Källén K & Bullarbo M (2014). Real-time PCR-assay in the delivery suite for determination of group B streptococcal colonization in a setting with risk-based antibiotic prophylaxis. Journal of Maternal-Fetal and Neonatal Medicing 27(4): 328-32.

Hansen R, Gibson S, De Paiva Alves *et al* (2018). Adaptive response of neonatal sepsis-derived Group B *Streptococcus* to bilirubin. Scientific Reports 8: 6470.

Hanson L, Van de Vusse L & Duster M (2014). Feasibility of oral prenatal probiotics against maternal group B streptococcus vaginal and rectal colonization. Journal of Obstetric Gynecological and Neonatal Nursing 43(3): 294-304.

Homer SE, Scarf V & Catling C (2014). Culture-based versus risk-based screening for the prevention of group B streptococcal disease in newborns: A review of national guidelines. Women and Birth 27: 46-51.

Hong J, Choi C & Park K (2010). Genital group B streptococcus carrier rate and serotype distribution in Korean pregnant women: implications for group B streptococcal disease in Korean neonates. Journal of Perinatal Medicine 38(4): 373-77.

Hughes RG, Brocklehurst P, Heath P *et al* (2003). Prevention of early onset neonatal group B streptococcal disease. London: RCOG.

Hughes RG, Brocklehurst P, Steer PJ *et al* on behalf of the Royal College of Obstetricians and Gynaecologists (2017). Prevention of early-onset neonatal group B streptococcal disease. Green-top Guideline No. 36. British Journal of Obstetrics and Gynaecology 124 :e280-e305.

Huttlinger Vigour T (2009). Mourning Sarah: a case for testing group B strep. Abingdon: Radcliffe Publishing.

Jamie WE, Edwards RK & Duff P (2004). Vaginal-perianal compared with vaginal-rectal cultures for identification of group B streptococci. Obstetrics and Gynecology 104(5 Pt 1): 1058-61.

Jao MS, Cheng PJ & Shaw SW (2006). Anaphylaxis to cefazolin during labor secondary to prophylaxis for group B Streptococcus: a case report. Journal of Reproductive Medicine 51(8): 655-58.

Joachim A, Matee MI & Massawe FA (2009). Maternal and neonatal colonisation of group B streptococcus at Muhimbili National Hospital in Dar es Salaam, Tanzania: prevalence, risk factors and antimicrobial resistance. BMC Public Health 9: 437.

Jones SM & Steel RW (2012). Recurrent group B streptococcal bacteremia. Clinical Pediatrics 51(9): 884-87.

Kaambwa B, Bryan S & Gray J (2010). Cost-effectiveness of rapid tests and other existing strategies for screening and management of early-onset group B streptococcus during labour. British Journal of Obstetrics and Gynaecology 117(13): 1616-27.

Kabiri D, Hants Y, Yarkoni TR et al (2015). Antepartum membrane stripping in GBS carriers, is it safe? (The STRIP-G Study). PLoS ONE 10:e0145905.

Kalin A, Acosta C, Kurinczuk JJ et al (2015). Severe sepsis in women with group B Streptococcus in pregnancy: an exploratory UK national case–control study. BMJ Open 5:e007976.

Kenyon S, Taylor DJ & Tarnow-Mordi W (2001). Broad spectrum antibiotics for preterm, prelabour rupture of fetal membranes: the ORACLE 1 randomised trial. Lancet 357: 979–88.

Kenyon SL, Taylor DJ & Tarnow-Mordi W (2001). Broad-spectrum antibiotics for spontaneous preterm labour: the ORACLE II randomised trial. Lancet, 357(9261): 989-94.

Khalil R, Uldbjerg N, Thorsen PB et al (2017). Risk-based screening combined with a PCR-based test for group B streptococci diminishes use of antibiotics in laboring women. European Journal of Obstetrics & Gynecology and Reproductive Biology 215: 188-192.

Khan MA, Faiz A Ashshi AM *et al* (2015). Maternal colonization of group B streptococcus: prevalence, associated factors and antimicrobial resistance. Annals of Saudi Medicine 35(6): 423-427.

Khan R, Anastasakis E & Kadir R (2008). Anaphylactic reaction to ceftriaxone in labour. An emerging complication. Journal of Obstetrics and Gynecology 28(7): 751-753.

Knight KM, Thornburg LL & McNanley AR (2012). The effect of intrapartum clindamycin on vaginal group B streptococcus colony counts. Journal of Maternal-Fetal Neonatal Medicine 25(6): 747-49.

Knudtson EJ, Lorenz LB, Skaggs VJ (2010). The effect of digital cervical examination on group B streptococcal culture. American Journal of Obstetrics and Gynecology 202(1): 58.e1-58.e4.

Kovavisarach E, Jarupisarnlert P & Kanjanaharuetai SJ (2008). The accuracy of late antenatal screening cultures in predicting intrapartum group B streptococcal colonization. Medical Association of Thailand 291(12): 1796-800.

Kozyrskyj AL, Bahreinian S & Azad MB (2011). Early life exposures: impact on asthma and allergic disease. Current Opinion in Allergy and Clinical Immunology 11: 400–06.

Kunze M, Zumstein K, Markfeld-Erol F *et al* (2015). Comparison of pre- and intrapartum screening of group B streptococci and adherence to screening guidelines: a cohort study. European Journal of Clinical Nutrition 69(6): 827-835.

Kwatra G, Cunnington MC, Merrall E *et al*, (2016). Prevalence of maternal colonisation with group B streptococcus: a systematic review and meta-analysis. The Lancet Infectious Diseases 16(9): 1076-84. doi: 10.1016/S1473-3099(16)30055-X.

Larsen JW & Sever JL (2008). Group B Streptococcus and pregnancy: a review. American Journal of Obstetrics and Gynecology 198(4): 440-50.

Lashkari HP, Chow P & Godambe S (2012). Aqueous 2% chlorhexidine-induced chemical burns in an extremely premature infant. Archives of Disease in Childhood: Fetal and Neonatal Edition 97: F64.

Le Doare K & Kampmann B (2014). Breast milk and Group B streptococcal infection: Vector of transmission or vehicle for protection? Vaccine 32(26): 3128-32.

Le Doare K, Allen L, Kiampmann B et al (2015). Anti-Group B Streptococcus antibody in infants born to mothers with human immunodeficiency virus (HIV) infection. Vaccine 33(5): 621-627.

Ledger WJ (2006). Prophylactic antibiotics in obstetrics–gynecology: a current asset, a future liability? Expert Review of Anti-infective Therapy 4(6): 957-64.

Lee B, Song Y & Kim M (2010). Epidemiology of group B streptococcus in Korean pregnant women. Epidemiology and Infection 138(2): 292-98.

Lin FC, Weisman LE, Azimi P et al (2011). Assessment of intrapartum antibiotic prophylaxis for the prevention of early-onset group B streptococcal disease. Pediatric Infectious Diseases Journal 30: 759-63.

MacDonald C, McLachlan R, Handorf S et al (2010). Group B Streptococcus: The impact of risk and prophylaxis on midwives and women in the childbirth experience. Birthspirit Midwifery Journal 6: 47-54.

Madhi SA, Cutland CL, Jose L et al (2016). Safety and immunogenicity of an investigational maternal trivalent group B streptococcus vaccine in healthy women and their infants: a randomized phase 1b/2 trial. The Lancet Infectious Diseases 16(8): 923-34.

Mavenyengwa RT, Afset JE & Schei B (2010). Group B streptococcus colonization during pregnancy and maternal-fetal transmission in Zimbabwe. Acta Obstetricia et Gynecologica Scandinavica 89(2): 250-255.

Mazzola G, Murphy K, Ross RP *et al* (2016). Early gut microbiota perturbations following intrapartum antibiotic prophylaxis to prevent group B streptococcal disease. PLoS ONE 11(6): e0157527.

McNanley AR, Glantz C, Hardy DJ *et al* (2007). The effect of intrapartum penicillin on vaginal group B streptococcus colony counts. American Journal of Obstetrics and Gynecology 197(6): 583-5.e1-4.

Money D, Dobson S, Cole L *et al* (2008). An evaluation of a rapid real time polymerase chain reaction assay for detection of group B streptococcus as part of a neonatal group B streptococcus prevention strategy. Journal of Obstetrics and Gynecology Canada 30(9): 770-75.

Morinis J, Shah J & Murthy P (2011). Horizontal transmission of group B streptococcus in a neonatal intensive care unit. Paediatrics and Child Health 16(6): 329-30.

Mueller M, Henle A, Droz S *et al* (2014a). Intrapartum detection of Group B streptococci colonization by rapid PCR-test on labor ward. European Journal of Obstetrics, Gynaecology and Reproductive Biology 176: 137-41.

Mueller NT, Whyatt R, Hoepner L *et al* (2014b). Prenatal exposure to antibiotics, cesarean section and risk of childhood obesity. International Journal of Obesity (London) 39(4):665-70.

Mueller NT, Bakacs E, Combellick J (2015). The infant microbiome development: mom matters. Trends in Molecular Medicine 21: 109-17.

Murphy-Lawless J (1998). Reading Birth and Death: A history of obstetric thinking. Cork, Cork University Press.

Neu J & Rushing J (2011). Cesarean versus vaginal delivery: Long term infant outcomes and the hygiene hypothesis. Clinics in perinatology 38: 321-31.

Nash C, Simmons E, Bhagat P *et al* (2014). Antimicrobial stewardship in the NICU: lessons we've learned. NeoReviews. 15(4): e116-e122.

National Institute for Health and Clinical Excellence (NICE) (2008). Antenatal Care. London: NICE.

National Institute for Health and Clinical Excellence (NICE) (2011). Caesarean section. London: NICE.

National Institute for Health and Clinical Excellence (NICE) (2019). Antenatal Care. London: NICE.

Neu J (2007). Perinatal and neonatal manipulation of the intestinal microbiome: a note of caution. Nutrition Reviews 65: 282–85.

Nguyen TM, Gauthier DW, Myles TD *et al* (1998). Detection of group B streptococcus: comparison of an optical immunoassay with direct plating and broth-enhanced culture methods. Journal of Maternal Fetal Medicine 7(4): 172-76.

NHS Choices (2014). Side effects of antibiotics. Available at: www.nhs.uk/Conditions/Antibiotics-penicillins/Pages/Side-effects.aspx

Oakley A (1980). Women Confined. Towards a sociology of childbirth. Cambridge: Martin Robertson.

Oakley A (1984). The Captured Womb. Oxford: Blackwell.

Oddie S & Embleton ND (2002). Risk factors for early onset neonatal group B streptococcal sepsis: case–control study. British Medical Journal 325: 308.

Odent M (2015). Group B streptococcal infection: beyond the mysteries. Midwifery Today 113: 12-13.

Ohlsson A & Myhr TL (1994). Intrapartum chemoprophylaxis of perinatal group B streptococcal infections: a critical review of randomized controlled trials. American Journal of Obstetrics and Gynecology 170: 910–17.

Ohlsson A & Shah V (2014). Intrapartum antibiotics for known maternal Group B streptococcal colonization. Cochrane Database of Systematic Reviews 2014, Issue 6. Art. No.: CD007467.

Ohlsson A, Shah VS & Stade BC (2014). Vaginal chlorhexidine during labour to prevent early-onset neonatal group B streptococcal infection. Cochrane Database of Systematic Reviews 2014, Issue 12. Art. No.: CD003520.

Olsen P, Williamson M, Traynor V *et al* (2018). The impact of oral probiotics on vaginal Group B Streptococcal colonisation rates in pregnant women: A pilot randomised control study. Women and Birth 31(1): 31-37.

Onderdonk AB, Delaney ML, Hinkson PL *et al* (1992). Quantitative and qualitative effects of douche preparations on vaginal microflora. Obstetrics & Gynecology 80: 333-38.

Onwuchuruba CN, Towers CV, Howard BC *et al* (2014). Transplacental passage of vancomycin from mother to neonate. American Journal of Obstetrics and Gynecology 210(4): 352-54.

Oster G, Edelsberg J & Hennegan K (2014). Prevention of group B streptococcal disease in the first 3 months of life: Would routine maternal immunization during pregnancy be cost-effective? Vaccine 32(37): 4778-85.

O'Sullivan CP, Lamagni T, Patel D *et al* (2019). Group B streptococcal disease in UK and Irish infants younger than 90 days, 2014–15: a prospective surveillance study. Lancet Infectious Diseases 19(1): 83-90.

Page-Ramsey SM, Johnstone SK, Kim D et al (2013). Prevalence of group B Streptococcus colonization in subsequent pregnancies of group B Streptococcus-colonized versus noncolonized women. American Journal of Perinatology 30(5): 383-8.

Paternoster M, Niola M & Graziano V (2017). Avoiding Chlorhexidine burns in preterm infants. Journal of Obstetrical, Gynecological and Neonatal Nursing. 46(2): 267-71.

Pelaez LM, Gelber SE, Fox NS *et al* (2009). Inappropriate use of vancomycin for preventing perinatal group B streptococcal (GBS) disease in laboring patients. Journal of Perinatal Medicine 37(5): 487-89.

Poncelet-Jasserand E, Forges F, Varlet MN *et al* (2013). Reduction of the use of antimicrobial drugs following the rapid detection of Streptococcus agalactiae in the vagina at delivery by real-time PCR assay. British Journal of Obstetrics & Gynaecology 120(9):1098-1109.

Rees JC (2014). Obsessive-compulsive disorder and gut microbiota dysregulation. Medical Hypotheses 82(2): 163-66.

Ross S (2007). Chlorhexidine as an alternative treatment for prevention of group B streptococcal disease. Midwifery Today 82: 42-43, 68.

Royal College of Obstetricians and Gynaecologists (RCOG) (2003). Prevention of early onset neonatal group B streptococcal disease: Green-top Guideline. London: RCOG.

Royal College of Obstetricians and Gynaecologists (RCOG) (2012). Prevention of early onset neonatal group B streptococcal disease: Green-top Guideline. London: RCOG.

Royal College of Obstetricians and Gynaecologists (RCOG) (2013). Group B streptococcus (GBS) infection in newborn babies. Patient Information leaflet. London: RCOG.

Sakru N, Inceboz T, Inceboz U *et al* (2006). Does vaginal douching affect the risk of vaginal infections in pregnant women? Saudi Medical Journal 27(2): 215-18.

Scasso S, Laufer J, Rodriguez G *et al* (2014). Vaginal group B streptococcus status during intrapartum antibiotic prophylaxis. International Journal of Gynecology & Obstetrics 129(1): 9-12.

Schrag SJ & Verani JR (2013). Intrapartum antibiotic prophylaxis for the prevention of perinatal group B streptococcal disease: experience in the United States and implications for a potential group B streptococcal vaccine. Vaccine 31(Suppl 4): D20-6.

Schrag SJ, Zell ER, Lynfield R *et al* (2002). A population-based comparison of strategies to prevent early-onset group B streptococcal disease in neonates. New England Journal of Medicine 347: 233-39.

Schuchat A (1999). Group B streptococcus. Lancet 353(9146): 51-56.

Seale J & Millar M (2014). Perinatal vertical transmission of antibiotic-resistant bacteria: a systematic review and proposed research strategy. British Journal of Obstetrics & Gynaecology 121(8): 923-8.

Seaward PG, Hannah ME, Myhr TL *et al* (1998). International multicenter term PROM study: evaluation of predictors of neonatal infection in infants born to patients with premature rupture of membranes at term. American Journal of Obstetrics and Gynecology 179: 635–9.

Seedat F, Geppert J, Stinton C *et al* (2019). Universal antenatal screening for group B streptococcus may cause more harm than good. British Medical Journal 364: l463.

Seoud M, Nassar AH, Zalloua P *et al* (2010). Prenatal and neonatal Group B Streptococcus screening and serotyping in Lebanon: incidence and implications. Acta Obstetricia et Gynecologica Scandinavica 89(3): 399-403.

Shore EM & Yudin MH (2012). Choice of antibiotic for group B streptococcus in women in labour based on antibiotic sensitivity testing. Journal of Obstetrics and Gynecology Canada 34(3): 230-35.

Sharpe M, Dennis K, Cates EC *et al* (2015). Deconstructing Dissonance: Ontario midwifery clients speak about their experiences of testing group B streptococcus–positive. Canadian Journal of Midwifery Research and Practice 14(2): 18-21, 28-33.

Singleton ML (2007). Group B strep prophylaxis: what are we creating? Midwifery Today 81: 18-20.

Slotved HC, Dayie NTKD, Banini JAN *et al* (2017). Carriage and serotype distribution of *Streptococcus agalactiae* in third trimester pregnancy in southern Ghana. BMC Pregnancy Childbirth 17: 238.

Spiel MH, Hacker MR, Haviland, MJ *et al* (2019). Racial disparities in intrapartum group B Streptococcus colonization: a higher incidence of conversion in African American women. Journal of Perinatology 39(3): 433-38.

Stapleton RD, Kahn JM & Evans LE (2005). Risk factors for group B streptococcal genitourinary tract colonization in pregnant women. Obstetrics & Gynecology 106(6): 1246-52.

Stewart CJ, Ajami NJ, O'Brien JL *et al* (2018). Temporal development of the gut microbiome in early childhood from the TEDDY study. Nature. doi.org/10.1038/s41586-018-0617-x

Stokholm J, Schjørring S, Eskildsen CE *et al* (2013). Antibiotic use during pregnancy alters the commensal vaginal microbiota. Clinical Microbiology and Infection 20(7): 629-35.

Stoll BJ, Hansen NI, Sánchez PJ *et al* (2011). Early onset neonatal sepsis: the burden of Group B Streptococcal and E. coli disease continues. Pediatrics 127(5): 817-26.

Sullivan SA & Soper D (2015). Antibiotic prophylaxis in obstetrics. American Journal of Obstetrics and Gynecology 212(5): 559-560.

Tajik P, van der Ham D & Zafarmand M (2014). Using vaginal Group B Streptococcus colonisation in women with preterm premature rupture of membranes to guide the decision for immediate delivery: a secondary analysis of the PPROMEXIL trials. British Journal of Obstetrics and Gynaecology 121(10): 1263-72.

Tam T, Bilinski E & Lombard E (2012). Recolonization of group B Streptococcus (GBS) in women with prior GBS genital colonization in pregnancy. Journal of Maternal, Fetal and Neonatal Medicine 25(10): 1987-89.

Tamma PD, Aucott SW, Milstone AM (2010). Chlorhexidine use in the Neonatal Intensive Care Unit: Results from a National Survey. Infection Control & Hospital Epidemiology 31(8): 846–49.

Towers CV, Howard BC & Onwuchuruba CN (2014). Vancomycin dosage for group B streptococcus prophylaxis. American Journal of Obstetrics and Gynecology dx.doi.org/10.1016/j.ajog.2014.06.040.

Trappe KL, Shaffer LE & Stempel LE (2011). Vaginal-perianal compared with vaginal-rectal cultures for detecting group B streptococci during pregnancy. Obstetrics & Gynecology 118(2/1): 313-17.

Tsakok T, McKeever TM, Yeo L et al (2013). Does early life exposure to antibiotics increase the risk of eczema? A systematic review. British Journal of Dermatology 169(5): 983-91.

Tse H, Wong SCY & Sridhar S (2014). Vancomycin dosage for group B streptococcus prophylaxis. American Journal of Obstetrics and Gynecology 211(5): 573-74.

Turnbaugh PJ, Ley RE & Hamady M (2007). The human microbiome project. Nature 449: 804–10.

Turrentine MA, Coliccia LC, Hirsch E *et al* (2016). Efficiency of screening for the recurrence of antenatal group B streptococcus colonization in a subsequent pregnancy: A systematic review and meta-analysis with independent patient data. American Journal of Perinatology 33(5): 510-17.

Turrentine M, Greisinger AJ, Brown KS *et al* (2013). Duration of intrapartum antibiotics for group B streptococcus on the diagnosis of clinical neonatal sepsis. Infectious Diseases in Obstetrics & Gynecology 2013: 525878.

Turrentine M (2014). Intrapartum antibiotic prophylaxis for Group B Streptococcus: has the time come to wait more than 4 hours? American Journal of Obstetrics and Gynecology 211(1): 15-17.

UK National Screening Committee (2008). Group B Streptococcus: The UK NSC policy on Group B Streptococcus screening in pregnancy. London: NSC.

UK National Screening Committee (2017). Group B Streptococcus screening in pregnancy. London: Public Health England.

Valkenburg-van den Berg AW, Sprij AJ & Dekker FW (2009). Association between colonization with Group B Streptococcus and preterm delivery: a systematic review. Acta Obstetricia et Gynecologica Scandinavica 88(9): 958-67.

Valkenburg-van den Berg AW, Sprij AJ, Oostvogel PM *et al* (2006). Prevalence of colonisation with group B Streptococci in pregnant women of a multi-ethnic population in The Netherlands. European Journal of Obstetrics, Gynecology & Reproductive Biology 124(2): 178-83.

Vergnano S, Embleton N, Collinson A (2010). Missed opportunities for preventing group B streptococcus infection. Archives of Disease in Childhood: Fetal and Neonatal Edition 95(1): F72-F73.

Vergnano S, Menson E, Kennea M *et al* (2011). Neonatal infections in England: the NeonIN surveillance network. Archives of Disease in Childhood: Fetal and Neonatal Edition 96(1): F9-F14.

Virranniemi M, Raudaskoski T, Haapsamo M *et al* (2018). The effect of screening-to-labor interval on the sensitivity of late-pregnancy culture in the prediction of group B streptococcus colonization at labor: A prospective multicenter cohort study. Acta Obstetricia et Gynecologica Scandinavica. https://doi.org/10.1111/aogs.13522

Wang LY, Chen CT, Liu WH *et al* (2007). Recurrent neonatal group B streptococcal disease associated with infected breast milk. Clinical Pediatrics 46(6): 547-49.

Watts G (2014). UK declares war on antimicrobial resistance. Lancet 384: 391.

Whitney C, Daly S & Limpongsanurak S (2004). The International Infections in Pregnancy Study: group B streptococcal colonization in pregnant women. Journal of Maternal-Fetal & Neonatal Medicine 15(5): 267-74.

Wickham S (2002). Epidural Fever. The Practising Midwife 5(8): 21.

Wickham S (2009). Screening and the consequences of knowledge. Birthspirit Midwifery Journal 2: 9-12.

Wickham S (2018a). What's Right For Me? Making decisions in pregnancy and childbirth. Avebury: Birthmoon Creations.

Wickham, S (2018b). Inducing Labour: making informed decisions. Avebury: Birthmoon Creations.

Yagupsky P, Menegus MA & Powell KR (1991). The changing spectrum of group B streptococcal disease in infants: an eleven-year experience in a tertiary care hospital. Pediatric Infectious Diseases Journal 10: 801-08.

Yancey MK, Schuchat A, Brown LK et al (1996). The accuracy of late antenatal screening cultures in predicting genital group B streptococcal colonization at delivery. Obstetrics & Gynecology 88(5): 811-15.

Zanetti-Dällenbach R, Lapaire O, Holzgreve W et al (2007). Neonatal Colonization-Rate with Group B Streptococcus is Lower in Neonates Born Underwater than after Conventional Vaginal Delivery. Geburtshilfe Frauenheilkd 67(10): 1114-19.

Zanetti-Dällenbach R, Lapaire O, Maertens A et al (2006). Water birth: is the water an additional reservoir for group B streptococcus? Archives of Gynecology & Obstetrics 273(4): 236-38.

Zhong H, Penders J, Shi Z et al (2019). Impact of early events and lifestyle on the gut microbiota and metabolic phenotypes in young school-age children. Microbiome. 10.1186/s40168-018-0608-z

Zilberman D, Williams SF & Kurian RR (2014). Does genital tract GBS colonization affect the latency period in patients with preterm premature rupture of membranes not in labor prior to 34 weeks?. Journal of Maternal-Fetal and Neonatal Medicine 27(4): 338-41.

Resources

I am aware that this book will be read by people in many different countries and that the structure of health services varies widely around the world. The amount of choice that people have also varies widely, not just because of regional geographical, political or economic differences, but as a result of income, education, ethnicity and other factors. This is absolutely not OK and I would encourage anybody who cares about the wellbeing of women, babies and families to read lots and get involved in creating awareness and change.

In an ideal world, every care provider would ensure that all women were fully informed about all of their options, rights and the possible pathways that they can take. Indeed, many women and families won't need or want to look further than their care provider for relevant information, which is great. So your care provider is a good first 'port of call', but some people will not yet have a care provider or may not feel that they have enough information from their care provider and will want to look further afield. Some women may have care providers who would like to help more but do not have the time, freedom or ability to do so.

These days, the internet is one of the best sources of information about women's birth rights on a local or national level. There are many groups, organisations and lists set up to share information online. In this appendix, I have included information for organisations that I know about and whose principles I know to be woman-centred. I would be happy to expand this list to include other organisations if anyone would like to send suggestions for inclusion in later editions of this book.

There are a few organisations which are specifically focused on women's birth rights. The best source of information about birth rights in the UK, for instance, is the organisation Birthrights (who can be found online at http://www.birthrights.org.uk/). They produce and update a whole series of factsheets on different topics which are available online. Another useful UK-based organisation is the Association for Improvement in the Maternity Services. AIMS' website is www.aims.org.uk and, in Ireland, AIMS Ireland offer resources, news and campaigning at http://aimsireland.ie/

In the US, Childbirth Connection offer information and factsheets at www.childbirthconnection.org/, including a useful leaflet entitled 'The Rights of Childbearing Women' which can be found at www.nationalpartnership.org/research-library/maternal-health/the-rights-of-childbearing-women.pdf

Often, pregnancy, birth, parenting or infant feeding related organisations run by women, birth workers (such as doulas, childbirth educators and breastfeeding supporters) and/or health professionals such as midwives and doctors can offer information, even if their primary focus doesn't quite match what you're looking for. A good example of what I mean by this is homebirth organisations such as Homebirth Australia (http://homebirthaustralia.org/) and Homebirth Aotearoa (https://homebirth.org.nz/). These kinds of organisations tend to be run by people who are very knowledgeable about women's rights and what is available within their country or area, even if you are not looking to birth at home.

If you are looking online for information, it can sometimes help to search for similar key words and phrases, for example, 'human rights', 'women's rights', 'reproductive rights' and 'childbirth rights'. Do search – both online and on local community noticeboards or gathering places - for local or national homebirth groups, doulas, childbirth educators, information on hypnobirthing, pregnancy yoga teachers and anything else pregnancy-related that you can think of. People who are interested in birth and related issues are often good at networking and sometimes you just need to find one starting point and then you'll have a way into lots of information. Don't forget parenting, postnatal and/or breastfeeding groups or supporters, postnatal yoga teachers and baby massage or similar groups. These are the people who have just been on the journey (or who support the people who have just been on the journey) and they can also be a good source of knowledge.

In some countries, home educators' groups, alternative community organisations or healthy living organisations can be a good source of support or information. Midwifery-focused organisations may also be a source of information, but this can vary a bit. Many countries have midwifery colleges or official organisations, but some of these tend to be focused on organising or regulating midwives. But there are a number of companies (like the US-based Midwifery Today magazine at www.midwiferytoday.com) and organisations (such as the UK-based Association of Radical Midwives at www.midwifery.org.uk) who will have websites and social media pages which you might find useful.

Inducing Labour: making informed decisions

Sara's bestselling book explains the process of induction of labour and shares information from research studies, debates and women's, midwives' and doctors' experiences to help women and families get informed and decide what is right for them.

Vitamin K and the Newborn

Find out everything you need to know about vitamin K; why it's offered to newborn babies, why are there different viewpoints on it and what do parents need to know in order to make the decision that is right for them and their baby?

What's Right For Me? Making decisions in pregnancy and childbirth

The decisions that we make about our childbirth journeys can shape our experiences, health and lives, and those of our families. A guide to the different approaches that exist; offering information, tips and tools to help you make the decisions that are right for you.

Birthing Your Placenta (with Nadine Edwards)

A popular book which helps parents, professionals and others to understand the process and the evidence relating to the birth of the placenta. No matter what kind of birth you are hoping for, this book will help you understand the issues and options.

101 tips for planning, writing and surviving your dissertation

These 101 tips are useful for students at any stage of their academic career. Written in an accessible, friendly style and seasoned with first-hand advice, this book combines sound, practical tips from an experienced academic with reminders of the value of creativity, chocolate and naps in your work.

Printed in Great Britain
by Amazon

84943357R00103